EMERGENCY DEPARTMENTS, JAILS, AND THE STREETS

Stories That Shaped My Career

Susan Laffan

Fulton Books, Inc.
Meadville, PA

Published by Fulton Books 2021

ISBN 978-1-63860-678-9 (paperback)
ISBN 978-1-63860-679-6 (digital)

Printed in the United States of America

To my mother and father, who taught me strong values; my husband, who always supported any decisions I made regarding my career; my children, Thomas and Katie, who put up with the crazy shift work and the times I was not home; and to my best friend, Debbie, who has been by my side through all this.

PREFACE

As 2021 will mark the fortieth anniversary of me being a registered nurse (RN), many people have said to me, "You should write a book," which is the inspiration for this book. I want to pay homage to those individuals whose lives I touched, even if they were never aware of it, to those who I have worked with, and for the support of my family and friends during each endeavor.

So the story really starts when I was in high school and I told my parents that I wanted to be a paramedic. Of course, I was influenced by the show *Emergency* back in the 1980s. I got accepted into the paramedic associate degree program right after high school, yet it was in Newark, New Jersey, and all classes where to be held in the evening. This did not thrill my mom at all since in the 1980s, it was not the safest town in New Jersey, especially after the sun went down. I told her of the time a guy followed me to my car, and before I could finish, she was about to tell me that "You are not going there anymore." I finished the story and told her it was the campus security guard who followed me to make sure I got to my car safely. I drove to Newark five evenings per week and every Saturday morning to fulfill my dream. About halfway through my training, I asked my parents if they thought I should switch to nursing because the paramedic program was still in the developmental stages in the States, and I did not want to graduate with a degree yet have no job to go to. I transferred my college credits and began my nursing degree. In August, before my last semester of nursing was to begin, the department head of the paramedic program contacted me and asked, "What have you been doing?" I told him I was finishing my nursing degree. He wanted me to come back to the paramedic program to finish my paramedic degree. You guessed it; I was going to nursing school during the day and paramedic school every evening for one semester. I graduated nursing school in December, took my nursing boards in February while attending didactic classroom sessions, practical in-hospital training, and four hundred hours of "riding time" by June of the same year. I completed my paramedic degree in May and passed my paramedic boards in June.

I have worked in some "normal" areas such as cardiac care unit, the emergency department (ED), post-cardiac catheterization unit, critical care transport, and some not-so-normal areas like county jails and nuclear power plants. My mom used to say, "I don't want to know where you are working next." I also rode as a volunteer on an ambulance in the town where I lived for about twenty years and worked as a full-time paramedic. In my spare time, while working full-time, I have also been an expert witness for lawyers nationwide, authored over forty articles, and have presented at state and national conferences for over twenty years. Add to the mix that approximately 85 percent of my nursing and paramedic careers were on the night shift. This could be a reason why, still to this day, my body does not want to sleep during the night.

Over the years, there have been some memorable stories, to say the least, some happy, some funny, some sad, and some tragic. Each encounter, I believe, helped me be a better nurse in one way or another.

Through much of this adventure has been my best friend, Debbie. We worked at many of the same places, and things just seemed to happen when we were there. We got through all of it one shift at a time. As you can imagine, there were many people whom I have worked with over the years. Some I can remember as if we worked together yesterday; some who I would like to forget, and some who I owe a world of gratitude to.

This book is formatted with stories that are grouped together according to different jobs or settings. Since I worked in many different emergency departments and various jails in New Jersey and other settings throughout my career, it would be impossible to put these stories in chronological order, and I am glad that my memory has retained all these stories over the years.

All patient names have been changed to protect their privacy and maintain confidentiality.

IN THE BEGINNING

Candy Striper at the Hospital

As I was in high school and determining what career I wanted to pursue, I signed up for the candy striper program at the local hospital. We would be assigned to assist with varying tasks such as delivering flowers and assisting with meal distribution to patients. One afternoon, I was tasked with bringing flowers up to the maternity ward that had just been delivered by local florists. That ward was on the third floor, and I would carry the flower arrangements up to the third floor two at a time via the stairwell. I became lifelong friends with one of the employees who worked in food services. Back in the day, a big meal cart would come from the main kitchen to each unit. The food service workers would place the food that the patient had ordered on a tray, and then the candy stripers would deliver the trays to each patient on that unit. This food service worker commented that my last name sounded familiar to her, yet we could not understand why since she had no children my age. She was older than me, and we did not attend any of the same places in town. After working with her for a few months, she told me she knew why my name sounded familiar. She said, "My husband replaced your father on the high school football team when your father graduated," and we had a laugh over that. We sent Christmas cards to each other for over thirty years. One year, I did not get a card from her and hoped it was just because she did not have my new address. The next year, I sent another Christmas card, and I received a letter in January from her husband. He had enclosed a memorial card and advised me that my friend had died of cancer. I cried when I received this news but was so grateful he sent me that memorial card because it is the only picture I have of my dear friend with her beautiful smile that would light up a room every time.

*****

This hospital had one of the only burn units in the state at this time, and I was assigned to that unit often. We were instructed that if there was an isolation sign and yellow tape on the floor to a room, we were not to go into that room and we would go tell the nurse that the patient's dinner tray was ready and the nurse would bring it to the patient after putting on gowns, gloves, and a mask. In a room almost directly across the hall from the kitchen where we prepared all the dinner trays, there was a man who had been severely burned over most of his body. He had been there for weeks in an isolation room, yet one day, when I came onto the unit, the isolation signs and tape were gone. I wondered if he had been discharged but learned that the same patient was in the room, yet he did not require isolation precautions anymore. I have to admit that I was nervous that I would have to bring the dinner tray into the man's room, not knowing what to expect. I did deliver his dinner tray, said hello, and only took a split-second glimpse of the patient, and I still remember to this day what that patient looked like.

Volunteer Ambulance Squad Before Becoming a Nurse and Paramedic

One of the prerequisites for the paramedic program is that you are already an emergency medical technician (EMT) and are volunteering with a first aid squad. So every Monday night from 6:00 PM to 6:00 AM, I was at the ambulance squad. We had one of those loud alarms like on the show *Emergency*. No sleeping through that! The ambulance squad was in the same building complex as the firehouse headquarters. One night, we did not have to travel far for the call of a fireman who was injured. While sliding down the fire pole from the second floor, he landed wrong and broke his ankle. I remember that night. I was on duty and stayed up late studying for my nursing boards that I would take over the next two days.

Nursing School

Not much happened in nursing school since it was a very controlled environment, where each student would only have one patient for a clinical block of time two days per week. I guess this was done for the best interest of the patients. One morning, I went into my patient's room, which was in bed A next to the hallway door. I was there to assist with his breakfast tray, and he only spoke Spanish. I introduced myself, smiled a lot, and we communicated by pointing to items on the tray. During this breakfast time, I heard an unsettling noise from the patient in bed B. I learned that the sound was what is called a death rattle. I went immediately to the nurses' desk and advised the other nurses. I returned to the room and started moving furniture out of the way since I knew what about to take place—a Code Blue. That patient did not survive, and I learned that day how fast things can happen.

*****

I was assigned to a toddler-aged child who was going to have a surgical procedure that day, and I had the task of giving the child an intermuscular injection. Before the procedure, my nursing instructor would accompany me, and when we arrived to the child's room, the mother asked me if I had ever given an injection before. My nursing instructor advised the mother that we had practiced this skill as nursing students yet told the mother that if she was uncomfortable with a student giving an injection, then we would have the primary nurse provide the task. The mother allowed me to give the injection and then told me that she thought I did very well.

*****

During another part of our pediatric rotation, we were going to a specialized children's hospital designed for children with developmental needs. We were each assigned one patient whom we would take care of from 9:00 AM to 1:00 PM for two days that week. Most of the children who lived there were awarded to the State and had no family who visited them, so the staff at the facility was very close to each of the patients. Each patient had a binder with all their medical information, their likes and dislikes, their nicknames, and their learning and mobility capabilities. My patient was a young boy would be turning ten years old the week after we were assigned there. I assisted the nurse getting the patient out of his pajamas and into the outfit for the day before breakfast. The challenge with him was that he had to be fed for each meal, and the food on the plate with different textures could not be mixed since he also had swallowing difficulties. I remember feeding him for breakfast, and it seemed as though time was racing away, yet I knew I could not rush him. After breakfast, we went back to his room, and I read him one of his favorite stories. I returned the next day to repeat the same tasks, and at the end of the day, my nursing instructor came to me to advise me that the facility staff nurse had commented on how well I did with feeding the child.

At the end of nursing school training, we were to have a big graduation ceremony at the college. I cannot remember if I was asked or if I volunteered to speak at our nursing graduation ceremony, yet I still have the original typewritten version of that speech.

Paramedic School

This learning environment was ever changing, and we responded to all kinds of calls and places. I did classroom work in Newark,

New Jersey, and "riding time" in Hackensack and Jersey City. My paramedic preceptors ranged from funny and helpful to stuffy and unwilling to teach. Since the paramedic program was in its infant stages of development, you were known or compared to other paramedics by your state certification number. When I was certified, my number was 497. The man who I would later marry was number 496. When we went out into the field with our preceptors, it was called riding time, which is different from clinical time in hospital units such as the emergency department, labor and delivery, EKG, and phlebotomy labs. I was assigned to ride with New Jersey paramedic certification number 2. I thought, *Wow! We got dispatched to a train versus an auto.* It was not far from the hospital and only took us about two minutes to get there. The train was stopped on the tracks in the middle of the crossing; and there was a mangled car against a telephone pole, and the firemen were on the other side of the train. No one could find the driver inside the car, so the search began to see if any occupants from the car had been ejected from the vehicle, all while having a train full of morning commuters looking on from inside the train and a very upset train conductor. The driver of the car was sitting on the side of the railroad tracks holding his index finger that had a laceration. He said when his car stalled on the tracks, he got out just in time. When we returned to the ER, the nurses were asking where the trauma victim was, and we pointed to the man holding his finger and said, "This is him."

*****

It had snowed all night, and everything was closed. The town tried to keep up with plowing the roads, but it was a losing battle. We got dispatched to an unresponsive twenty-year-old. We were going to this call on a highway overpass with two lanes each way, chain link fences on either side, and two highways—Route 17 and Route 80—underneath, about sixty feet below. There was no traffic on the roads, thank goodness, but we started to slide down the overpass sideways, and all I could think was that the fence will not stop us from falling.

The driver got control, and we arrived to find a twenty-year-old who had overdosed many hours before in the basement of the house. The police were there and asked us what we thought happened, and we pointed out the suicide note and empty bottle of pain pills on the floor. His mother said his girlfriend broke up with him, so she took him to a bar the night before.

*****

While riding in Jersey City, we got dispatched in the early hours of the morning to a motorcycle crash in the Holland Tunnel. I said to the paramedic, "I've never been in the Holland Tunnel," and his response was "Well, you're going tonight." You know things are bad when on a weekend night, you arrive to the inbound (to New York) tunnel lanes and there are just a sea of brake lights and there are no cars coming out of the outbound lanes. Well, we went in the open lanes and just kept going. If you have ever been in the tunnels between New Jersey and New York, you know that on the wall, there is a marking to advise you what state you are in. We traveled and were about fifty feet from that marker. A motorcycle had struck a box mail truck head on. The motorcycle operator, approximately 350 pounds, was on the road in the tunnel with his helmet still on, but his femur was obviously broken, and he was very restless to the point of being agitated. We had no communication with the radios being that far into the tunnel, so we could not advise the hospital of this patient. He had a passenger who was on the side of the road holding her wrist. The motorcycle operator had an obvious fractured femur but also had, as we would learn later, a traumatic tear in his aorta. The police told the hospital staff that his wife was on her way to the hospital, so they turned to the girl who was on the motorcycle and asked her who she was.

She said, "His girlfriend."

After the call, the paramedic said to me, "I wonder what he hit."

I said, "Didn't you see the box truck?"

"No," he replied.

"You were leaning against it when we were getting the guy on the stretcher," I said.

*****

One of the first cardiac arrest calls I was on as a student was a test of all I had learned regarding safety of defibrillation. The patient was an overweight man who collapsed in one of the smallest kitchens I have ever been in. He need to be defibrillated, so the paramedic who had the paddles in his hands charging handed them to me and said, "Go for it." In that split second, I thought of all lessons I had been taught. *Do not stand over the patient. Do not stand in any liquids. Do not touch any metal and apply enough pressure to the paddles to the patient's chest so the electric current does not arc from paddle to paddle.* It was a challenge since the man was surrounded by water that he dropped. The only spot I could stand was almost against the metal refrigerator, and all of us were in that tiny kitchen. Well, I did it and vowed to myself that I would never hand "live" paddles to anyone like that, and I am happy to say I never did.

*****

One hot spring Friday night in Newark, New Jersey, at the newly opened University of Medicine and Dentistry, I was to go for my first ER shift rotation as a paramedic student. At the time, this was the only trauma center in the state. They had two large resuscitation rooms, and I got to see both of them in action that night. During the course of the evening, we received two hanging victims from two separate jails. The first male was a tall, muscular man who succumbed to his attempt. The second male was a small lightweight man who survived. It was a sign of things to come in my career, even if I did not know that at the time.

I had some great paramedic preceptors in the field that took the time to show me the ropes and hoped that one day I might do the same for new paramedics. I did not want to be like the paramedic instructors that felt students were an inconvenience to them or were not willing to share their knowledge and experience with students. I was lucky to only have one such paramedic that was not happy with the preceptor task.

Nursing: Progressive Care Unit (PCU)

My first job as a new registered nurse was on the progressive care unit because when I went for the interview, I told them that I was also a paramedic, so I knew how to start IVs, and I could read a cardiac monitor. The nurse who interviewed me and hired me turned out to be one of the night-shift supervisors when I worked in the ED years later. I got a job in the hospital where my paramedic career was to begin, but the program was not starting until October. I got hired in June to work in the progressive care unit with the understanding that once the paramedic program started, I would later transfer within the hospital. I was the only registered nurse on that unit, working with other licensed practical nurses (LPNs) each night. To this day, I remember the RN who oriented me to the floor and the LPNs who guided me through the transition from student to "real" nurse. Not only did I have to hang all IV medications, flush all IVs, I had to mix them also. So each night, I would have to go through the medication cart to make sure I had all the medications for the midnight doses. After two weeks on this unit, I became the relief charge nurse on the night shift.

After working in the cardiac care unit (CCU) at another hospital, I transferred to the progressive care unit (PCU) at this hospital. Our unit was directly one floor up from the emergency department. Things were different back in the day as far as security goes. Our unit had approximately thirty rooms and sixty patients when full, and we were almost always full. Back then, any ventilator patients stayed in the hospital because there were no facilities that could take care of long-term ventilator patients. We had a patient on our unit for months. I believe he suffered a stroke and was ventilator-dependent.

He was unresponsive, and the family had a caregiver with him on the overnight shift. She did not do nursing care, yet she could reposition him and just be there to keep him company. One shift night, I was in charge, and I was also the medication nurse. This patient's room was a private room right across from the nursing desk, which was in the middle of the hall of all the patient rooms. I was at the far end of the hallway hanging an IV medication and heard a blood-curdling scream. I ran out of the room and saw someone come from this patient's room run across the hall and down the stairwell that lead to the emergency department and outside. I ran down the hall and found the caregiver in the room, visibly upset, and I asked her what happened. She stated that she just went to the break room for a minute, and when she returned to the room, a man was by Mr. Jones's bed with a plug in his hand. She said that was when she screamed, and he ran out. I checked the patient first, heard that the ventilator was still functioning, and no alarms were going off. I checked the electrical outlet near the head of the bed to see what plug had been pulled out. It was the cord for the bed controls. I called the nursing supervisor, who came to the unit, and after I told her what I knew, she said, "Why didn't you go after him?" My first thought was to say because my profession is a nurse, not a police officer or security guard, but I just said that I went to check the patient's well-being immediately. Well, the police came and took statements, and the family was notified. For the next few days, we had a security guard posted outside Mr. Jones's room. The investigation revealed that the man was a dear friend of the family who referred to Mr. Jones as Pop. He told the police that he could not stand to see Mr. Jones like that anymore and wanted to just pull the plug. Mr. Jones never improved from the devastating effects the stroke left him with, and after many months on the unit, he died.

*****

In one report, I was told that we might get a transfer from a Florida hospital. Because of the long travel distance, they were not sure when Joe would arrive at our hospital in New Jersey. Joe was a twenty-two-year-old male who grew up in the town where this hospital was located. The nurse aide who worked on our unit said that the name sounded familiar, and she thought she went to high school with Joe. He graduated and moved to Florida where he was going to college. Joe attempted suicide when his girlfriend left him by taking a loaded gun to his right temple and pulled the trigger. He survived the traumatic event, yet his family wanted him close to home to recover. Joe did arrive in the middle of the night by ambulance. His head was shaved on the right side where a craniotomy had been performed. He had a feeding tube and a urinary catheter. After we moved him into the bed, we decided to give Joe a bath from head to toe because he had such body odor from the long ride, and the remainder of his hair was all matted. Joe had a temperature of 101 degrees. He had no skin breakdown, no drainage from the surgical site, which was already healing. I decided that the urinary catheter should be changed since the collection bag had so much sediment in it. A specimen of the urine was sent to the lab. Joe would open his eyes yet did not speak, did not follow commands, yet it seemed like he could understand what we were saying. Since Joe was young and so were all the nurses working that night, I called the emergency department to see if a male nurse could come replace the urinary catheter. When the old catheter was removed, on the balloon that keeps the catheter in place was a big white fuzzy thing growing on it. We sent that to the lab also. Then it came time for the bed bath, so the nurse aide and myself pulled Joe to the head of the bed, put a basin under his head, and gave him a long shampoo, then a bath, and he looked so much better. His family came every day to visit him while he was on the unit, during the daytime. Joe was supposed to be transferred to a long-term care facility, yet every time he was medically cleared to go, he would spike another fever, which was protocol to delay the transfer until the cause of the fever was determined and treated. We knew that physical therapy worked with Joe during the day hours, yet each night, we would go into Joe's room and do range of motion exercises, talk to him, show him magazines of cars, and turn him to prevent bedsores. At one point, we had Joe holding a magazine with assistance. I honestly think he was more awake during the night shift than any other time of the day. We did not want Joe to lose any more muscle tone or get complications such as foot drop, and if he could hear and more importantly understand us, we wanted him to know that we cared about him. The nurse aide did recognize Joe from high school, and one day, Joe looked right at her and gave this mean grimace. I am not sure if he recognized her from high school or if she reminded him of his girlfriend. We knew Joe was again cleared to be transferred that day, and we told him that "if you want to get out of here, do not get a temperature." I looked at Joe, and a tear was rolling down his face. That just melted my heart because I really felt he could hear and understand at least part of what we were saying. Many years later, while I was working in the emergency department, I got a report that a patient Joe with a history of a craniotomy after a gunshot wound was sent for a fever from a rehabilitation facility. After getting the report on all the patients in the emergency department, I had to go see him. His family was next to him.

His mother said, "I don't know why they send him here all the time for a fever. He has been through so much." "He doesn't even know we are here."

I introduced myself and told the mother that I was the nurse on duty the night Joe got transferred back to New Jersey. She thanked me and all the other staff team members for all that we did while Joe was in the hospital. I had to fight back the tears while talking to her because Joe had severe contractures to both arms and legs, was pale and thin, and was now a shadow of who he was before.

*****

Since I was the nurse who had recently graduated, I was the person who would document on each patient's chart their updated nursing care plans. Back then, we did not have computer-generated templates, so they were all handwritten. I had to be creative when a patient was on the unit for any length of time, yet I actually loved doing these.

This progressive care unit was moving to a different floor in the hospital, right next to the cardiac care unit, which made sense, since patient coming from that unit came to PCU. We arrived for our 11:00 PM–7:00 AM shift and were just getting a report when the doors flew open with a patient, with a terrified look on her face, in a hospital bed in severe respiratory distress being pushed by three nurses from another nursing unit.

"What room? What room?" They were yelling. We pulled a bed out of one of the patient rooms and called a Code Blue.

The hospital operator announced, "Code Blue PCU, Code Blue PCU!"

While waiting for the house doctor, respiratory therapist, nursing supervisor, and CCU nurse assigned to respond to Code Blues, we had to start chest compressions and ventilate the patient. Yet nobody came to help us. We called for another Code Blue.

Once again, it was announced, "Code Blue PCU. Code Blue PCU!"

My charge nurse knew that I was a paramedic and said, "Why don't you intubate her?"

I told her that since I am working as a nurse in a hospital, I cannot legally perform duties of a paramedic. The unit phone began to ring. It was the respiratory therapist asking, "Where are you guys now?" None of the other hospital staff members had been notified that the progressive care unit was moved to a different location on the day shift. They all arrived within a minute after the phone call to assist us, and the patient was moved to the CCU for further treatment.

Nursing: Emergency Departments

We were a very tight-knit "family" back in the day. Working the night shift, your world is opposite everyone else's. As paramedics, we would work, talk, and socialize with doctors, nurses, firemen, and police officers. After working years as a paramedic, one night, I came into the ER with a patient, and the charge nurse on the night shift, who had been there for many years wanted to talk to me. She said that she was retiring and that she wanted me to be the new charge nurse on the night shift in the ER. She knew I was also a nurse. She realized I knew all the ER staff, and I guess she thought I was the best one for the job. Remember, back then, there were not only RNs but also LPNs working in the ER, and she told me that none of the other RNs wanted to be in charge. I considered it, and eventually did move into the ER as the night charge nurse. To this day, the people I worked with remain close to my heart, although sadly, some of them have gone to heaven. We truly were like a family. We worked in an area that was a resort area during the summer. We would get so busy in the summer months, and then as September came around, things would get to normal. Each year, we would have an end-of-summer party. We would all bring food, laugh, tell stories, and just relax. We would have Christmas parties also and any other excuse to have a get-together. We enjoyed the birth of new children, children growing up, those who got engaged, and those who got married. We bonded together when tragedy struck—such as, a death or an accident that affected one of our crew or one of their family members. The few times when the ER was not going crazy, we would enjoy listening to the rain outside and watching lighting storms while sitting outside in wheelchairs with either soda or coffee. Police officers would visit the ED and bring us doughnuts and just check up on us. The pace was different back then, and we now know how valuable those times were.

While working in emergency departments, there are some phrases seasoned nurses would never say such as "it is quiet in here" and "I have seen everything now." The emergency department is a unique place in the hospital. Things can change literally in an instant and go from calm and controlled to crazy and insane in a matter of minutes. The night shift was always staffed with fewer personnel, and many times, we needed extra help get through those crazy times. I would like to think that working in a hospital was safe, yet at times, people did get out of control. We were lucky that not all the hospital security guards were of retirement age and could be of help to us if someone got out of control. As I was at the main nursing desk for the emergency department, a woman came from the treatment area screaming, "I am going to get my money's worth out of this hospital!" Our hallway outside the x-ray room had chairs lining the wall for patient's waiting for x-rays to be taken. That hallway led down to the main x-ray department, and there was a treatment room to the left off that hallway. The lady proceeded to go down that hallway screaming the entire time as people on those chairs began to get out of the hall. She stopped midway down the hall and tried to tear a phone off the wall. When she could not get it off the wall, she continued to scream and head down the hall to the x-ray department. During this time, one of the other staff members had called the local police on what we referred to as the "bat phone," which was a direct line from the emergency room to the police dispatcher. The police arrived, went down the hall to the x-ray department, and put the woman in handcuffs and escorted her out. As the patient returned to their seats in the hall, one patient said, "Boy, that was something," and I answered, "You should see Friday nights. We sell tickets."

*****

As I was coming from the treatment area back to the nurse's desk, I heard a man yelling, "I want a drink of water!" I saw the man standing at the nurse's desk, with an open pocketknife waving it at the nurse at the desk. As she backed away from the man, unbeknownst to her, I reached for the "bat phone." The police responded and escorted the man out of the emergency room. The nurse turned to me and said, "I am not sitting there anymore."

*****

A patient came to the ED with the complaint that an object was stuck in his rectum. After the physician examined the patient and removed the object, he wrote discharge instructions. Keep in mind that this was in the early 1980s, before computer-generated instructions. As I went to have the patient sign the discharge papers, I saw that the physician wrote, "Avoid fruits and vegetables."

*****

It was another hot summer night, and the ED was packed with people waiting to be seen. There were patients admitted to the hospital who would have to hold in the ED overnight since there were no hospital beds available. This was very common in our ED, and the ED staff would have to take care of admitted patients as well as any new patients arriving. The three-to-eleven-shift charge nurse gave me a report that there was a homeless man in the lobby who had been there for hours. They told me to call the police if he became a problem, and they would return and arrest him for vagrancy. As I said, the ED was crazy busy that night. We had a young boy and his mother in our bereavement room being treated. The homeless man started getting loud and begging people for money in the lobby, so we called the police whom I thought had already knew of this situation based on the three-to-eleven shift report. All of a sudden, we could see numerous police cars heading toward our doors with their lights flashing, wondering what was going on. The K-9 officer and dog came through the door as the young boy with his mother yelled, "Look, Mommy, the police dog!" I met him a few feet from the door and asked him what was going on, and he said, "You called us." I explained it was for the homeless man in the lobby, so the police left the ER, taking the man with them.

*****

On another night, the police brought in someone who was under arrest and had to be medically screened before going to jail. It was another busy night that we had people in all treatment areas and stretchers lining the hallways. They put the patient and officer in the cast room since that room had a door, and it would keep him away from other patients. The officer handcuffed one arm of the patient to the stretcher and waited to be seen by a doctor. As I was down the hall trying to start an IV on a frail old woman who needed a blood transfusion, I heard a large bang. One of the other nurses went to see what was going on and came back yelling, "Susie, we need help!" The cast room door was closed, and we could not get it open. Another nurse was in the room with the patient and police officer trying to help. The patient had flipped the stretcher upright while still handcuffed to it and was trying to get to the officer's gun. Sometime during this event, a visitor of the patient had gotten in the room also. When we all got the situation under control, I looked at the visitor, who was on the floor, and said to her, "Weren't you here last week for an overdose?" They both got medically cleared and went to jail that night.

*****

Another patient who was in her third trimester came in for a nosebleed. The husband came up to the nursing desk and yell out, "You people are as useless as tits on a bull!" He was threatening and yelling at all of us, and the ED physician came from the treatment area and yelled, "Who is yelling at my nurses?" This husband caused ongoing problems any time his wife came to the ED so much so that he was told he would not be allowed into the ED if his behavior did not change. He threatened us with lawsuits and harm. We had so much respect and love for our physician who would stand up to people like this and watch out for our safety.

*****

There were times when patient outcomes were wonderful. Such is the case with a forty-year-old man who came in to the ED in cardiac arrest. We worked on him for what seemed to be forever, and two hours later, while still being in the ED awaiting transfer to the CCU, he was sitting up on the stretcher, still on a ventilator, writing notes to the nurses and his family on a pad of paper. He thanked the staff for saving his life, and the family could not give us enough hugs while they were crying tears of joy.

It is hard to work in the ED on holidays because not only are you away from your family, but bad things always seem to happen to those who should be celebrating. Examples of this are when mothers die on Mother's Day, fathers on Father's Day, people who die on or near a holiday, anniversary, or birthday. As nurses, we stay with the families after the doctors advised them that their family member is no longer with us. This can be draining on the nurses since we are there to support and comfort them, try to answer any questions, and realize that the gift of life is out of our control no matter what we do. I cannot tell you how many people have said things like "Next week is our fiftieth anniversary," "His birthday is next week," and "Christmas will never be the same," to mention a few.

It is also hard to work in an ED in the area where you live because you realize people you know can come or be brought to the ED at any time. I was at home one evening about 5:00 PM, scheduled to work that night at 11:00 PM when my phone rang. It was one of the paramedics calling me to tell me that our beloved unit secretary, who was in her late twenties, was brought in as a cardiac arrest. I threw my uniform on and sped to the hospital. They were still doing CPR on her when I arrived. After trying to revive her to no avail, she was pronounced dead. Everyone was in shock from the doctors to the nurses to the paramedics, and all the other ED staff. I had to perform the difficult task of calling each of the night-shift staff members and telling them this extremely sad news. Those who were scheduled to work needed to know before they got to work, and those who were off needed to hear it from me. Each of them could not believe what I was telling them, and one nurse told me many, many years later that she thought I was drunk when I called, yet she knew I did not drink alcohol. Many of the staff came in just to lend support to one another. Some of the three-to-eleven-shift nurses told me they would stay over if anyone from my shift was unable to come in that night. I would find out later that it was a berry aneurysm that caused her death. She had a smile that could light up any room, and I know we all miss her dearly.

During another night shift, we were told that our unit manager's husband was being brought to the ED in cardiac arrest. Another night, a staff doctor was being brought to the ED in cardiac arrest. Once again, we poured everything we had into their care and treatment, and once again, neither of them survived.

There really were good times sprinkled into all the tragedy and death we saw and had to deal with. One year, we decorated the ED with paper snowflakes and hung them from the ceiling. We also had Boy Scout troops make pictures for what Christmas meant to them. We hung them in the ED lobby where people could view them and put a sign up that said "Christmas through the Eyes of Children."

*****

When I was very pregnant and still working, I was at the nurse's desk and happened to look at the EKG recordings of those on cardiac monitors. All of a sudden, a patient went into ventricular fibrillation (V-fib), so I took off running into cardiac 1 and yelled for help. I was moving so fast that I actually slid into the side rail of the stretcher, and the patient looked at me and said, "Is anything wrong?"

I glanced at the monitor, and she went back into a normal rhythm. I said, "No, nothing is wrong."

She asked me why so many people were in the room. I turned around, and almost all the nurses working that night were in the room. I said to her, "See how good they are when I yell?" I told the doctor what had happened. He reviewed the EKG strips that had recorded it and were lying next to the central monitor. He was a bit surprised and then put her on a medication to prevent similar episodes.

*****

A ninety-six-year old lady was brought to the ED for having what she called a spell. The nurse assigned to that section was busy, so I went in to get the patient chart started. I changed her into a hospital gown, put her on the cardiac monitor, took her vital signs, and asked her questions about her medical history and medications, while the ED technician did a 12-lead EKG. I went back to the nurses' desk to start typing in the information of the chart when I looked at the cardiac monitors and saw the patient's heart rate went from being in the seventies to the twenties. I ran to the room and found the woman unresponsive with a weak pulse of twenty. I grabbed the equipment needed to assist her in breathing when I heard one of the two ED doctors now in the room said, "Is that for real?" I said yes and put the head of the stretcher down to assist her ventilations, and all of a sudden, her heart rate came back up into the seventies. It was determined that she needed a pacemaker to help her heart through these spells, as she referred to them. After she was stable, the ED doctors said to me, "We have never seen you move that fast, so we thought we both better follow you." We all got a chuckle out of that statement.

*****

A young man came into the ED complaining that he could not breathe. He had a laceration to his upper back and told us that he had fallen off a ladder. His color was very pale. His skin was moist, and his vital signs revealed that he was going into shock. A portable chest x-ray was done and revealed that he had a hemothorax (blood in his lung). The ED doctor had to put in a chest tube to alleviate the pressure being put on his lung and drain the blood. He tolerated the procedure well and was stable awaiting transfer to the intensive care unit when a police officer arrived and said he needed to speak to the patient. It was discovered that he was actually stabbed by a broken beer bottle during a fight with another male.

*****

Another night, we had a pedestrian struck by a car on a bridge. This bridge went from the mainland to the barrier island and resort town on the Atlantic coast. The paramedics attempted to revive him, yet he had sustained massive internal injuries when the car struck him, and he was thrown into the air before landing on the pavement. When he arrived to the ED to be transferred to the morgue, other than being very pale, he had no visible injuries. His family was contacted and were present in the ED when I got a phone call from one of the hospital security guards who said that he had a young lady that was hysterical in the hospital main lobby screaming that she wanted to see her boyfriend. I told the security guard to bring her to the ED. When they arrived, the family recognized her. The young lady continued saying, "I have to see him, and I am not leaving here until I do." The family gave permission for her to see him, and she said that she had a fight with him earlier, and the last time she saw him was when she left him on top of the bridge.

*****

During the night, the paramedics responded to a car that struck a tree. The paramedics had provided pre-hospital care, yet the patient died at the scene. I was told by the paramedics that he had massive head injuries, revealing brain matter on the sheets mixed in with the blood. He was brought to the morgue. About an hour later, I received a phone call from the local police department asking questions about the patient. There was concern that the identification that was found with the patient may not have been his. They wanted to know if the patient who came into the ED had a scar on his thigh since the person whose identification was found had surgery with a stainless-steel rod surgically placed for a fractured femur in the past. The local police officers said they wanted to go see the patient, and I advised them that he had already been moved to the morgue. When they arrived, we all headed to the morgue. I knew that they would not want to see the massive head injury, and I did not want any of them fainting or vomiting in the morgue. When we got to the morgue, I told them all to turn their backs to the patient while I unzipped the body bag. Honestly, I did not want to see that head injury, so I unzipped the body bag and put a towel over the patient's head. They saw what they needed to investigate and left since the patient did have an open fracture to the lower thigh. Later in the night, another officer came in, and I told him what we had to do, and he said, "I knew he had a rod in his leg because when they were taking pictures at the scene, I saw the rod when they used the camera flash."

*****

We had a pregnant female arrive to the ED in active labor. It was policy that the ED physician had to examine the patient before going to the labor and delivery unit. As soon as she got on the stretcher, she screamed, "The baby is coming now!" She delivered a healthy baby girl within three minutes after arriving to the ED. We had to call the nursery and told them we have a new baby in our Isolette. A labor and delivery nurse, a nurse from the nursery, and the respiratory therapist came to the ED to transfer them up to their unit, later to be discharged without complications.

*****

While working in the ED one night, we received a phone call from one of the medical floors. They had a patient who was experiencing an allergic reaction, and her tongue was swelling. The house doctor was not able to protect her airway with intubation, and they wanted the ED doctor to go to the floor, yet he was the only doctor in the ED. The house physician had to come to the ED before the ED doctor could go to the floor. This happened quickly, and the next phone call the ED received was the floor nurse stating that the ED doctor wanted me to go to the floor immediately to help him. I ran to the elevators since the ED was on the first floor, and this medical unit was on the fourth floor. Not to waste time, and I was young at the time, I headed up the stairwell. As I hit the fourth-floor landing, I heard a Code Blue being announced over the public address system for that unit, and upon my arrival, I knew exactly what room I was going to since, from down the hall, I could see furniture being thrown out of a room into the hallway. I knew the respiratory therapist, nursing supervisor, and a nurse from critical care unit would be responding as they were assigned to respond to any Code Blues in the hospital. Another nurse from the ED arrived, and the doctor said to us that he was going to have to do an emergency tracheotomy since her airway was already closed to attempt intubation. The patient was awake, with terrified eyes looking at us, gasping for any breath. The three of us worked together, the doctor doing the tracheotomy with the assistance of the other ED nurse and respiratory therapist while I monitored the patient's heart rate. The patient's heart rate dropped into the thirties. I advised the ED doctor and was already opening the box of atropine and giving the proper dose IV as he said, "Give it." Her heart rate went up. The tracheotomy was in place, and the patient's condition was improving. The nursing supervisor already had an intensive care bed available for the patient to be transferred. We all returned to the ED after the event on the fourth floor and were exhausted. Weeks later, the ED doctor asked me if I got a copy of the letter he wrote and gave to the ED nurse manager. Neither the other ED nurse nor I knew anything of what he was talking about. He brought us each a copy of the letter a few nights later, and it was him thanking us for assisting him in saving this patient's life.

*****

When salmonella poisoning affects someone, they usually have massive bouts of foul-smelling diarrhea, dehydration, and fever. We had five people come to the ED with salmonella poisoning from food they had eaten earlier during the day. We had an observation room, with a door, that had three stretchers, so we adapted it to accommodate five stretchers and placed them in that room. The entire night, all we did was provide IV fluids, empty bedside commodes numerous times while dealing with the rancid smell from their diarrhea. We could not wait to get home that morning and each take long hot showers.

*****

One April night, one week before Easter was just crazy in the ED. There were no in-patient telemetry or critical care beds in the hospital. When our shift started, we were already holding admitted patients on cardiac monitors. We were using all wall-mounted monitors and all portable monitors and, at one point, had to get other portable cardiac monitors from storage in the hospital. As if this shift had not seemed like it went on forever, approximately at 5:30 AM, we got a patient in cardiac arrest. While working on that patient, another patient came in with severe respiratory distress who needed to be intubated. We had moved two patients out of our trauma room so these two patients could receive care and that all the ED nurses and the two ED doctors could be in one room working together for these two new patients. While in the middle of this, the paramedics went running out of the ED yelling, "Baby code!" I had to quickly decide where this baby code was going to go to get treatment. We moved a patient out of the cardiac room and pulled the pediatric code cart from the trauma room into the cardiac room. About two minutes later, the paramedics returned, and I thought, *Oh, good, it is not a baby code.* The paramedics then said the police were already on their way in with the baby doing CPR. Just as the paramedic ended this sentence, I saw the headlights and red lights of the police car heading straight toward the ED doors. The two policemen working on this infant were also both paramedics. The ED unit secretary, who was witnessing all this chaos, knew that a staff pediatrician came to the hospital every morning at 6:00 AM to do hospital rounds. She called the pediatric unit and explained what was happening, and the pediatrician came down to provide care to the child, so the ED physicians could remain with the other two critically ill patients. The day-shift nurses began to arrive, some around 6:30 AM to have their morning coffee and get prepared to start their shift, and they took one look at my face and realized something was wrong. All I could say was that "There are three patients who are not on cardiac monitors. There is a code going on in trauma 1, and a severe respiratory distress being intubated in trauma 2, and a pediatric code in cardiac 2."

One said to me, "Finish what you are doing, I will figure the rest out."

The elderly man in trauma 1 died. The middle-aged man in trauma 2 was intubated and going to be admitted to intensive care unit, and the child in cardiac 2 also died. I stayed with the family of the child giving support, finishing up documentation, and my shift that night ended at 9:00 AM.

*****

One early morning around 5:00 AM, a patient was brought to the ED with a broken ankle. She was in her midforties and had obviously been drinking alcohol by the smell of her breath. After the first aid squad moved her onto the ED stretcher, I uncovered her ankle to get a look at this fracture. It was an open fracture (fracture with an open wound), and her foot was almost turned around to face the wrong way. I tried to find a pulse in her foot to verify adequate circulation. I found a weak pulse, put an *X* to mark the location and tried to support her foot and ankle in a position where she would not lose that pulse. The x-ray technician came over to do a portable x-ray because we could not chance moving this patient on and off an x-ray table. I had to stay in that room holding the patient's foot and lower leg until we could get it wrapped and splinted in such a way that would maintain pulses in her foot. Surprisingly enough, the patient did not even complain of pain and tried to get off the stretcher a few times. Her blood alcohol came back, and she was found legally intoxicated. The dilemma came as to when she would be legally sober to sign an operative consent and safe to have the surgery. I never saw an extremity being held together by just skin and a small amount of muscle like that. My shift ended, and eventually she went to surgery later that day.

*****

An ED doctor was in talking with a family about the condition of their father when the patient went into cardiac arrest. I went to advise the doctor that we needed him to see a patient, and he responded, "I will be there shortly." I did not want to say in front of the family members that it was their father in cardiac arrest, yet I had to get the doctor to the bedside of this patient. I said to him, "I need you right now." The family asked me if they could go see their father now, and I told them I would be back to get them shortly. The doctor was not happy that I interrupted him. Until we got out of earshot of the family, I told him what was going on. We provided care, and the patient survived. Then the ED doctor went back and explained what had happened to the family so they could be at his bedside.

*****

Sometimes the staff in the ED remains the same for long periods, yet there are always times when people transfer to different departments or change jobs altogether. New staff may have experience working in an ED, and some are relatively new to this environment. I was standing at one end of the nurse's desk one night when a patient's clipboard came flying by me and hit the desk. I turned around, and it had been thrown by one of the doctors new to this ED. He said sorry, and I went over to him and explained that he was not to throw things around. Of course, I said it in a rather motherly way. We laughed about it today, yet I was ready to wring his neck at the time.

*****

Back in the day, before trauma centers were designed, our ED leaders decided to initiate a new protocol called a trauma alert. It was intended to notify via the hospital operator over the entire hospital's overhead announcement system key personnel that a trauma victim was coming into the ED. This included the x-ray department, the laboratory that was supposed to bring non-crossmatched blood to the ED, the operating room and staff, the nursing supervisor, the chaplain, social workers, any surgeons in the hospital at the time, and ancillary staff such as security. The theory behind it made sense, yet for the night shift, it really was not going to help us much. We did not have an operating room open after 11:00 PM. There was no chaplain or social workers. There was only one person in both the laboratory and x-ray departments, and no extra physicians in the hospital. I brought my concerns to the medical director, and he said that it could not be changed or adapted just for the night shift. A few weeks later, we had a trauma patient coming in with the paramedics around 1:00 AM. I followed the protocol and called the hospital operator and told her we needed a trauma alert called. She asked me what that was. I quickly explained to her to announce it over the intercom system. Anyone who has worked in a hospital on the night shift understands that the only time there is an announcement over the intercom system was for a Code Blue. Usually the operator would announce the Code Blue in a normal tone advising those responding where the Code Blue was taking place. When I hung up the phone, the announcement came over the intercom system, yet the operator was yelling it out, and it was so loud. The telephone lines in the ED lit up like a Christmas tree, and all the calls were from staff members working in the hospital asking us, "Is it a boy or a girl?" "What happened?" "How old are they?" and "Where are they coming from?" They were all concerned about family members, yet this tied up all our phone lines, and cell phones were not available then. We could not even make an outside phone call if we needed to. After this event, I spoke with the medical director again, and he agreed that all we needed to do was page or call the nursing supervisor, security, the laboratory, and the x-ray department working on the night shift.

*****

We got a report that a physician's son was involved in a car accident and trapped in the vehicle. Paramedics were on the scene, and the fire department was trying to extricate the young man from the car. This was about 10:00 PM. We notified the operating staff, which was soon to go off duty. The news of this spreads like wild fire, and we had all kinds of doctors responding to the ED, including the patient's father, the urologist. They were gathered in the ED, saying, "Where are they? What is taking so long?" The ED doctor explained that paramedics were on the scene and already treating him while he was being extricated from the car. When he arrived, he already had intravenous lines and had received fluids. The ED doctor examined him. We got the necessary x-rays completed, monitored his vital signs, and inserted a Foley catheter, and he was off to the operating room. He was in the ED for approximately fifteen minutes before going to surgery. He survived the trauma to his body, came through surgery well, and went to intensive care, then the step-down unit, to a regular floor before being discharged. The patient's father weeks later bought food and thanked the OR staff, ICU staff, progressive care staff, and surgical floor staff in appreciation for the wonderful job they did for his son. He never mentioned the paramedics or the ED staff. Later on that night, as if that wasn't enough for us, we received a call from the county dispatcher center that there was a fire in town, and there may be hazardous materials burning and that we may receive patients from this fire. It turned out that since they did not know what was burning inside the barn, the county medical doctor deemed it necessary that all the EMTs who were at this fire had to come to the ED to be checked out with a chest x-ray and an arterial blood gas drawn to check for carboxyhemoglobin. A short time later, approximately at 1:45 AM, an ambulance was backing up to the ED doors. When the ambulance doors opened, there had to be about twenty people inside the ambulance coming to be checked out. Then they told us a few more ambulances were transporting more people. We had a nurse at the ED door, and if they had no symptoms or respiratory distress, they went to the lobby to have their vital signs taken and make an ED chart. We recruited two other first aid squads who were not at the fire to do the vital signs for us. There was one young lady who had some wheezing and a history of asthma, so she was placed directly on an ED stretcher and taken care of. We made a line from the lobby after the chart was made. They went to x-ray, then sat in the hall to have their arterial blood gas drawn. Keep in mind that we had other ED patients in the ED at this time. We had a computer ordering system, yet that system went to *downtime* each night at 2:00 AM. When in downtime, requests slips had to be handwritten to complete the order. We had it under control, yet around 3:00 AM, the medical director of the ED arrived and told me that "Help is on the way." By the time the day-shift nurses arrived, all the patients had their tests done and were just waiting to be seen by the county doctor. The only problem with a computer downtime is that any orders that were requested on those handwritten slips then had to be put into the system as a late entry once the downtime was completed. The night shift was used to this routine since it happened every night, yet I was there for a number of hours putting in all the late-entry orders once the downtime was completed. That night felt like it would never end, only to find out that the medical director had breakfast brought in at 7:45 AM thanking those who came in to help. The night shift had already clocked out by that time, and we were never advised that breakfast was on the way.

*****

Since our hospital was near the famous Jersey Shore, the summers could be super busy. The town itself had approximately one hundred thousand residents, and countless numbers of people would come to the shore each summer. One summer in particular, we had so many motor vehicle accidents between Memorial Day and Labor Day that when Labor Day weekend approached, I said to the nursing supervisor that if we had any fatalities from motor vehicle accidents, then she would have to come down to the ED and comfort the family. The ED night staff had seen so much tragedy that summer we could take no more. Some of the saddest accidents involved young people. There was a lot of alcohol involved and speeding on the highway that connected the Garden State Parkway to the Jersey Shore. The gridlock of cars on Saturday mornings heading east to the shore and the cars going west on Sunday night made residents try to avoid that road at all costs during those times. There was one accident in which two brothers were in a car that struck a tree, and they both died. Another accident was a young female who was driving her car and got struck by a car that went through a red light and killed her. The most tragic part was that her parents were in the car behind her and saw the whole event and were devastated.

*****

One morning, around 6:30 AM, we received an elderly woman from a nursing home for altered mental status. The ED technician and I went to get her into a hospital gown, put her on a heart monitor, and get an EKG. While we were leaning her forward to get her nightgown off and I was going to listen to her lungs, we found the cause of the altered mental status. The patient was ordered fentanyl patches for treatment of pain that was routinely ordered, "Apply one patch every seventy-two hours." I looked at her back, and she had six fentanyl patches on her back, which we quickly removed. She was not in any respiratory distress, so she was observed and monitored in the ED then returned to the nursing home with discharge instructions to remove fentanyl patch when a new patch is applied.

*****

Our hospital had a policy that if you called out sick on a recognized holiday, you would be written up and reprimanded. On the night shift, we rarely had this issue, and the staff was very accommodating toward one another especially during the Christmas to New Year holidays. The other shifts seemed to always have issues with staffing. It did not matter what holidays you worked on my shift as long as it did not cause overtime and that the proper staffing levels were met. I was the night charge nurse when I was pregnant and had my first child. Since my husband also worked the night shift, most of my babysitters were staff that worked in the ED at the time. On

Christmas Eve, my babysitter called me and had to cancel because of the flu. I know she would never do this unless she was truly sick. With no family nearby and the knowledge that I would be written up if I did not go to work, I packed my child up in his pajamas, and off we went to work. This was in the time when we were not crazy in the ED on a typical night and usually very slow on a holiday. We got a crib and placed it in the observation area, which was right in front of the nursing station. It was a quiet night, yet none of us would ever say those words. About halfway through the night, I saw the nursing supervisor heading down the hallway toward the ED. This was something she would do every night. If she did not come down early in the shift, then we knew there had to be issues going on in other areas of the hospital that she had to deal with. She came up to the nursing desk and looked around and said, "At least it is a good night for you now on Christmas Eve." She turned to see the young boy in the crib and said, "Ahh, too bad he is here on Christmas Eve." Then she realized that there was no parent at this child's bedside and looked at me.

I said, "Well, I could not call out," and she realized that it was my son. As she turned to leave the ED, she said "I do not know anything." When my son woke up around 5:30 AM, he received Christmas presents that the staff had brought in for me to give to him later that morning, so we all had a Merry Christmas while he opened his gifts.

*****

Working in the ED of the town where you live and where my husband is a police officer and paramedic and where my best friend Debbie's brother is a police officer and paramedic can put added stress to the night. One night, Debbie and I were both working in the ED, and my husband and Debbie's brother were also working as police officers when we heard a call for shots fired. Both our hearts sank at that moment, and there was nothing we could do but listen to the police radio for any information about who the police officer was and what was going on. Those few minutes were the longest time in my life, while the ED staff prepared the trauma room just in case. The dispatcher who was stationed in the ED in a room called Medcom called the police department to get any information and advised them that both Debbie and I were working that night. I remember hearing him say, "They already know something is happening out there." It turned out to be that another officer who was involved with someone who was trying to assault him and get his weapon, and the shots fired was the police officer's way to let the other officers know where he was since he was in the middle of a field at this point and nowhere near his police car. The officer was visibly shaken up and brought to the ED to be evaluated by the doctor. I did not know that Debbie asked the police officer for his gun so she could lock it in the narcotic cabinet until the investigators would arrive. So when I asked the officer where his gun was, he told me that "I gave it to Debbie." All I could say was "Are you crazy?" and it did help lighten the moment. Even though the town had a big population, there were not many shots-fired calls back in the day.

*****

I was sleeping with my infant son home one night when there was another shots-fired call in town, and this time, it involved my husband. The paramedics raced out of the ED heading toward the scene, and Debbie wanted to go with them, yet she was told she could not. So Debbie called her mom, who is also a nurse, paramedic, and rides on the volunteer first squad to let her know what was going on, and Debbie asked her mom if she could go to my house to watch my son if needed. Just prior to all this, a police officer from a neighboring town was getting assaulted, so most of the officers from our town were on the opposite side of town from my husband assisting that officer. Apparently, my husband saw a suspicious vehicle come out one of the car dealerships and attempted to make a motor vehicle stop. At one point, the driver of the stolen car started heading toward my husband to hit him with the car. The only way my husband could stop the car was to shoot into the car engine, which disabled the car but not before the car had struck my husband. Meanwhile, back in the ED, they all waited for any news or updates. Debbie told the staff that if I had heard what was going on via the scanner, then I would have called or come to the ED by now. My husband never went to the ED to get checked out. Debbie's brother apparently drove by my house numerous times throughout the night and in the morning to see if we were all right. I knew nothing of this whole event until two days later when I saw the large bruise on my husband's leg and asked him where he got it from. His reply was simply "When the car hit me the other night." Well, that is when the questions began, and I learned of the whole event.

*****

It was a slow night in the ED and the first county sheriff K-9 was on patrol with his handler. The officer would stop in to the ED every now and then just to chat and see how we were all doing. One night, I asked him if I could see his K-9, whose name was Attitude. I just loved that name for this muscular German shepherd. He said sure, and we all went out to the ED's parking lot. The sheriff officer was Hispanic and spoke English and Spanish, yet Attitude only responded to commands in German. He took Attitude out of the car and told us not to approach him yet. He gave Attitude some commands in German and told us we could come and pet him. We played with him for a bit, and then the officer told us to go back and stand by the ED doors. He gave Attitude another command and told us to come on back. The minute we took one step, that dog was ready to attack and barked like crazy. We ended the meet and greet with Attitude on a good note and were able to give him a treat.

*****

We had a middle-aged female patient come into the ED with a very rapid heart rate and began to get symptomatic with low blood pressure and pale skin. The doctor ordered adenosine IV push, which is a drug used to block receptors in the heart and convert the irregular rhythm back into a normal rhythm and rate. The drug is given intravenously fast push of one to two seconds and flushed immediately so the entire dose gets in the circulatory system. When you give this drug, be prepared because most patients' heartbeat may stop for a few seconds. I was aware of that, yet I was not prepared for when I gave the medication, and she let out a loud scream, then her heart rate stopped as the ED doctor, myself, and the other ED nurse watched the cardiac monitor. After only a few seconds, her heart rate returned and went to a normal range in the eighties. She was a bit groggy, yet later said to me that she actually "felt the medication hit her heart." She was the only patient who had ever screamed or told me that is what the medication felt like.

*****

Since we could only hold so many admitted patients in the ED overnight, and there was just not enough room or extra hospital beds to accommodate them, the staff on the night shift would almost, on a nightly basis, get egg crate cushions, cut them to fit the ED stretchers, make the "bed" up, and transfer all the admitted patients onto these "beds." Finding pillows for ED patients had always been a challenge because pillows seemed to get swallowed up on the in-patient units. We would send the housekeeper up to the floors to find pillows for all our patients so we could make them as comfortable as possible. For a stretch of over two weeks, we were holding anywhere from two to fifteen cardiac monitor patients overnight in the ED, awaiting transfer to in-patient beds. Every morning, the day shift would come in and begin their day with all these admitted patients and pending transfers. All of a sudden, one night, we had no holding patients to pass on to the day shift. So it was time to have a little fun. We each put on a portable cardiac monitor, so the main cardiac monitor screen showed we had patients on monitors once again, yet we closed all the curtains to the patient stretchers. As the day shift

41

reported for duty, they were tired to start another shift thinking there were many holding patients. Psych!

✦✦✦✦✦

When I was the night charge nurse in the first ED I worked in during the 1980s, nurses' week was approaching. Typically, we all wore a specific color scrub uniform for each unit in the hospital. I always wondered why as a nursing student I had to wear a white uniform when taking care of patients, yet that was the normal. Most of the ED nurses were older than me and came from various locations. We decided that for nurses' week, we would wear our nursing caps to work. It was not feasible to wear a white uniform in an emergency department. The other shifts made fun of us, but we did not care. Our ED served a large elderly population, and I cannot tell you how many people commented on how professional we looked. When they would ask us why we were doing this, we responded that we were celebrating nurses' week, and many people thanked us for all that we do.

Over the many years in this ED by the Jersey Shore, we had so many people come in that were intoxicated, from young teenagers to the elderly. Treatment cannot be based on the blood alcohol number but by the symptoms presented. A teenager could come in and have a blood alcohol laboratory level of 100 (1) and be knocked out; whereas, an alcoholic could be walking around maybe with unsteady gait with an alcohol level of 400 (4). Getting intoxicated patients was almost a given, especially during the summer months. The ED staff made up a game called guess the level. We had to guess the patient's alcohol level as they arrived to the ED just by looking at them. We would write the bets down and wait for the laboratory results. For some reason, the person who was always the closest to the actual number was our unit secretary.

We had a homeless man in town who drank alcohol, and the ambulance squads and paramedics were dispatched to pedestrian-struck calls numerous times throughout the year. Motorists would be upset or think they struck the man with their car, yet in reality, it

EMERGENCY DEPARTMENTS, JAILS, AND THE STREETS

was Jack, who was intoxicated and fell off his bicycle or just fell down by the road.

*****

Nurses typically have one particular area they like, and one they just hate. I always loved the emergency department, yet labor and delivery was the area that I never liked nor never worked in. Some nurses are just not a correct fit for the ED. Back in the 1980s, after you took your nursing board examination, it could be weeks to months until you heard the score. You were to work as a *graduate nurse*, which meant you had restrictions on some of the tasks that you could perform, such as starting or giving any medication through an IV site. In those days, you were required to have experience working in as a nurse before being hired to work in the ED, yet a graduate nurse was assigned to work in our ED. Let us just say that it was a bad choice, and numerous events occurred that were or could have been avoided.

*****

There were times when we were expected to get large amounts of snow in New Jersey. Most times, arrangements could be in place for other personnel to pick up staff in vehicles that could handle better in the snow. One time, I had to wait over thirty minutes in the blizzard conditions to get picked up, and when I arrived to work, my hair, even though it was covered, was frozen. There were times though that *essential personnel* would be out of the pickup zone, so we would stay over at the hospital. I remember sleeping on a stretcher in the same day at a surgery area during one snowstorm and sleeping on a cot set up in a conference room during a different snowstorm.

43

Nursing: Nuclear Power Plant

My friend Debbie recruited me to work at the nuclear power plant about fifteen miles from our town. They were hiring nurses to be there around the clock during an *outage*. The reactors were not shut down, yet it was the time all different contractors come in to do repairs on the plant. Everyone had to go through dress-in-dress-out protocol in case you had to go into the reactor area. They instructed us that there are lines painted on the floor indicating *hot spots*, and anything else is the green zone. We also had to do random drug testing and breathalyzer testing on the workers and respond to any medical emergencies in the plant. A name that was picked at random by a computer would come off the printer, and we had to contact that person's supervisor that they had to come to medical within thirty minutes of the name printing out. Sometimes the person was not working that shift or had not yet arrived for their scheduled shift. During training, we practiced doing these tests and the procedure to follow if a positive result came up. My first night working there, a name printed, and I notified the supervisor of this contractor. The supervisor told me the contractor was scheduled to arrive at 8:00 PM. At approximately 8:10 PM, the man arrived to the medical unit, and we proceeded on with the testing. When we got to the breathalyzer test, after he blew into the machine, it just kept cycling and cycling, and I thought that it never took this long when we were practicing. Just then the value came on the screen, and the value represented legally intoxicated. I could not believe this for my first one. I followed the protocol and called the head of the medical department as well as his supervisor. After his supervisor arrived, we had to repeat the test on a different machine, and the result was the same.

The gentleman said to me, "I was drinking earlier today, but I thought it would be out of my system by now."

Having a positive result equates to immediate termination.

*****

It had been a record-setting heat wave in New Jersey with the daytime temperatures being over one hundred degrees for days. The low temperature at night would not go below ninety degrees. The medical unit was outside the actual power plant yet within the confines of strict security. I was in the medical unit when both the phone and the radio went off at the same time for a man-down-in-the-reactor call. The caller told me that a security guard would escort me to where the patient was. All I kept thinking was *Let him be in the green zone away from the line of contamination.* I had to go through the security screening x-ray, put on my hard hat, and off into the huge building with mazes for hallways we went. As if ninety-eight degrees outside was not hot enough, inside was worse. We finally arrived to the elevator and went down a few flights. When the doors opened, I could see someone sitting on a chair with his head down and a crowd of people around him. With the light behind him and the mist, it looked like something from the movie *Flashdance* when the dancer was working as a welder. The staff EMTs escorted me over to the man, who at this point, only had on boxers sitting on a chair. The contamination line was about twenty-five feet from me, yet the man had not been in the hot zone, so we did not have to put on all the protective gear. The man was obviously in heat exhaustion, so we had to get him out of this area.

Just then the EMT whispered into my ear, "We have a problem. The elevator we came down in is not working."

We did not know when and if it would be working again, so I told all the workers to each grab a leg of the chair the man was sitting on and told them we were heading toward the stairs. I stayed behind them so I could watch the man in case his condition changed. We had to take frequent breaks going up the stairs. At one point, the man looked like he was going to vomit, so I stopped them from moving, took the man's hard hat off, and put it in his lap. We then continued up the stairs and out of the building. When we got outside, even though it was close to ninety-five degrees out, it still felt wonderful. We went into the medical unit and laid the man down and put cool cloths on him initially. Once he was feeling better, he was able to take fluids. He did go to the hospital for an evaluation but was released by morning.

Nursing: Critical Care Transport

The company that I worked for had a critical care transport crew composed of two EMTs and a registered nurse, and they had equipment and medication similar to what was in a crash cart on a hospital floor and additional medication that could be used during the transport if needed. We would transport patients via an ambulance from one facility to another. Examples of critical care transports included trauma patients from an ED to a trauma center, patients being transferred to a stroke center, pediatric patients going to a pediatric specialty hospital, patients going for a cardiac catheterization, and anyone who needed cardiac monitoring, a ventilator, or intravenous fluids or medication or both during the transport. We would be notified after the sending facility had already contacted the receiving hospital and the patient was accepted and that there was an available bed for that patient. We would frequently transport patients to various trauma centers and specialty hospitals or units.

The theme for any busy night was the song "Just Another Manic Monday" by the Bangles. We would call those who would not move out of the way of the ambulance Jack, yet we felt we should have a name for a female, so we called them Jill. I was at an expansive outdoor market one time, and I saw a person who made signs from letters off license plates, and don't you know? There was one for both Jack and Jill. I did not buy them, yet I sent a picture of them to the EMTs whom I worked with for a laugh.

On one call, we were transporting a patient to one of those trauma centers, and when we got one block from the trauma center, there were police cars everywhere. We did not know, nor were we notified of what all the police activity was about. We brought our patient to their assigned unit, and then upon leaving the hospital, we found out that there had been a shooting inside the lobby of the emergency department's waiting room. A few weeks later, I spoke to the charge nurse of the ED and voiced my concerns about us entering into a potentially dangerous environment. We discussed the hospital's protocol for these types of disasters, and I suggested that they should build into their protocol to notify various dispatchers, so they would be able to advise any ambulances heading to that hospital what was going on.

*****

During one of our northeast storms, the winds and rain were getting progressively worse as the night went on. We were dispatched to transfer a stroke patient from an ED to a stroke center. Our protocol was to call the stroke center when we were fifteen minutes away so the stroke center could activate a Code Stroke, and all the assigned personnel would be present when we arrived. The woman was already on a ventilator and had been unresponsive since we arrived in the ED. Her eyes already had a gaze to the left, and her pupils were nonreactive, these both being very ominous signs. We transferred the patient to our stretcher, connected our ventilator, and headed out into the crazy weather.

We were traveling on an interstate highway, and the driver of the ambulance said, "The wind is blowing us all over the road."

I told her to take her time and get us there safely. As this was happening, the patient's blood pressure was rising higher and higher. We already had physician orders to treat this scenario, and I called the stroke center to give the receiving nurse an update. I was trying to draw up the medication with a syringe from a vial as we continued to slide from one lane to another because of the wind. Her blood pressure was getting dangerously high, yet I took one more blood pressure prior to giving the medication I now had ready to administer. Within one minute from the last blood pressure reading, she dropped her blood pressure almost in half before I gave the medication. We called the stroke center when we were fifteen minutes away and arrived only to have the lights in the hospital go out about ten seconds after we arrived. The generators went on, and we continued to the CAT scan suite where the stroke team had assembled.

The receiving nurse looked at my monitor and saw the current blood pressure and said, "It dropped too fast."

I explained that I had not given any medication, and we all knew that this patient had a very grave prognosis.

One of the doctors asked us, "How is it out there?" and we said bad. He questioned, "Why are you out there then?"

My response was "because the stroke center had accepted the patient, and we were the only way the patient would get here." Shortly after that, the Office of Emergency Management shut all bridges from New Jersey to Philadelphia because of high winds.

*****

We were transporting a man in his late fifties from an in-patient telemetry (heart monitor) unit to a hospital in Philadelphia for a cardiac catheterization. He had gone to the hospital with complaints of chest pain hours before. We arrived on the unit. I received report from the assigned nurse, and we went into the patient's room to introduce ourselves and prepare the patient for transport by placing him on our cardiac monitor and took his vital signs. Of course, he was anxious about the catheterization, which is understandable, yet it appeared that something else was wrong. I asked the patient if he currently had any chest pain, and he replied no. I asked him if anything else was bothering him.

He said, "I have a massive headache."

A nitroglycerine patch had been applied earlier, which was not to be removed, yet one of the common side effects of nitroglycerine is that it gives patients a headache since all the blood vessels in the body are opened up or dilated. As my crew made the patient comfortable on the stretcher, I went back out to the nurses' station and asked the assigned nurse if the patient had received any Tylenol while on the unit. When she replied no, I asked her to please administer Tylenol to the patient before we transport him since he had a headache. I think she was a bit annoyed, yet I explained to her that Tylenol is not a medication we carry on the ambulance, and I was hoping to reduce or alleviate the patient's headache prior to arriving at the receiving hospital. We waited while the nurse gave the patient the Tylenol, then we were on our way. About twenty minutes into the transport, as my patient and EMT were talking about sports teams, I asked him how his headache was.

He responded, "It is almost gone. Thanks."

Those are the small yet important feelings of accomplishment when, as a nurse, I can be an advocate for the patient, and they feel better as a result.

*****

We were to transport an infant to the specialized children's hospital approximately forty minutes away. The infant was brought in for lethargy and was found to have a low blood sugar. The ED doctor seemed unsure that this infant could be transferred without the specialty hospital's transfer team. I was receiving report from the pediatric ED nurse when the ED doctor came over to me and said, "Can you take a blood sugar reading during the transport? Because if you cannot, I will have to call the specialized transport team." I assured the doctor I could and would do a blood sugar reading at the time increment they wanted. I then asked the ED doctor for any orders to have based on the blood sugar reading—such as, if the level is below a certain number, then give a certain dosage of medication (glucose), and if the level was high, was there an order to reduce the intravenous infusing rate? The ED doctor wrote the orders on an order sheet, and we added that to the chart already prepared for transport. I did the blood sugar reading at the time specified, and it was within the normal limits, so no other medication had to be given or adjusted. The transport went smoothly, and the patient was transferred to the care of the specialized children's hospital ED staff. I decided to call the sending ED doctor just to advise them of the transport, the blood sugar level, and that no other medications had to be given or adjusted. The ED doctor seemed relieved that the transport went well.

*****

We were often dispatched to be *on standby* at hospital's cardiac catheter labs that could not provide open heart surgery, should the patient need that intervention. We would get a general report from the nurse taking care of the patient, either in the ED or on an in-patient unit. Working the night shift, most of the cardiac catheter labs were closed, and the team had to respond to the hospital to do the procedure. My crew and I were already at the hospital's cardiac catheter lab awaiting both the team and patient who was coming from an in-patient floor. All of a sudden, a hospital bed came around the corner with a patient on a cardiac monitor. The patient went into cardiac arrest in the hallway as the cardiac catheter team was setting up the cardiac catheter lab. My team and I moved the patient into the cardiac catheter lab, moved him onto the procedure table, and began doing chest compressions. The patient regained a cardiac rhythm so the cardiac catheter team began their procedure. This was a special call because for both EMTs working with me that night, it was the first time they did CPR on a patient, and the patient regained a cardiac rhythm, which medical professionals refer to as a save.

*****

Our transports could be from five miles long to over three hundred miles long, depending where the patient was being transferred to. The two farthest transfers I had were that of a patient who was being transferred to Baltimore, Maryland, one night, and two weeks later, I got dispatched for a patient going to Washington, DC. Both transfers were from central New Jersey. We had a patient who had extensive abdominal surgeries in the past and had to be transported back to the hospital that had done all the surgeries. The transport was going to take a few hours, and the ED physician had the patient medicated for pain just prior to our arrival. The ED nurse told me that the patient had received pain medication a few times while in the ED. I asked the ED doctor for a one-time order for pain medication since the transport was going to be lengthy. He agreed and gave me a written order for a one-time dose of pain medication. We were only in the ambulance about twenty minutes when the patient asked for pain medication. I reminded him that he had just received pain medication prior to leaving the ED and that I had a one-time medication order. I explained to him that we should hold off for some time. That way, if the pain got worse later in the trip, we could medicate him appropriately. The patient asked me what medication did the doctor order, and I told him it was Dilaudid, then the patient asked me for the dose, and I told him that it was 2mg and given intravenously. The patient had been on pain management after the abdominal surgeries and was aware of the different medications used for pain control. We began to talk about various topics from sports to jobs to hobbies. The patient then took a nap as we continued to the receiving hospital. Later in the transport, the patient once again asked for pain medication, and I administered the Dilaudid as ordered. The patient thanked me for listening, and that waiting for the pain medication to be given was the right choice.

*****

The transport RN would get a text on her assigned phone with any assignments for that shift. As we were heading to the sending facility, the RN would call for report. Sometimes we would not get much of a report prior to arriving simply because the assigned nurse was busy with the patient, getting them prepared for the transport. If the assigned transport RN had a critical patient with numerous tasks to be completed or monitored, they could ask our dispatchers to have another RN accompany them with the patient. It was company policy that all patients on cardiac balloon pumps had two RNs on the transport—one to monitor the balloon pump and one to monitor the patient. I was dispatched to go with another RN and crew to transport a critically ill young female going to a hospital approximately two hours away, barring no traffic. We headed out and arrived to the receiving hospital with the patient who was going to the intensive care unit. I had trained as a paramedic in this hospital when it first opened approximately thirty years before. After we moved the patient into the assigned bed, as the transport RN gave the report, I looked around the unit.

One of the EMTs asked me, "What's wrong?" based on my facial expression, I guess. I realized this was the very same intensive care unit I trained in and was remembering some of the patients who were in this very same unit thirty years prior. I remembered the man with a massive head injury after being struck in the head with a baseball bat, the man who lost part of his upper leg because of a train accident, and the time there were two families fighting in the intensive care unit waiting room, and the ICU staff were instructed to barricade the doors so they could not get into the unit as we heard people hitting the wall next to us.

*****

We would sometimes have to transport a newborn, yet this involved more than just our crew. We would have to go to the receiving facility, pick up their transport team that consisted of a pediatrician, nursery RN, and a respiratory therapist. We would have to leave our stretcher at that facility and load the Isolette into our ambulance. These calls seemed to take a long time because there were discussions among doctors, nurses, respiratory therapists, and parents to name a few, before we could even get to the actual transport. We would all head back to the receiving hospital, and we would pick up our stretcher and go in service for the next call.

*****

Coordination, communication, and timing between all staff involved are the key to a smooth transport. We were positioned in various areas of the area hospitals we covered. As requests for transfers came in to our communication office, the dispatchers had to activate the most appropriate crew to each call. We were to transport a patient with an ascending aortic aneurysm (AAA) to a helicopter landing zone about four miles away that was located on the grounds of another hospital affiliated within the same hospital system. We arrived to the sending hospital, got report, and loaded the patient on to our stretcher. Because of the patient's diagnosis, which could be lethal if the aneurysm bursts, I did not want to be sitting in a parking lot awaiting a helicopter if this occurred. I had the ED unit secretary call hospital security at the hospital with the landing zone to ask if the helicopter had landed, and it had not as of yet. I explained to the ED doctor and RN that I would be waiting until the helicopter was in sight of an approach before I was going to transport, and they understood my rationale. The patient was already moved to our stretcher and placed on our monitoring equipment, and we had his chart in hand. We received word that the helicopter was overhead the landing zone, so we headed that way. The transfer of patient to the flight crew and helicopter was uneventful, and the patient was flown to the receiving hospital for repair of the AAA.

*****

We arrived at an ED that had a patient being sent to a trauma center, and the ED staff advised me that the trauma center RN needed to talk to me. The trauma center RN asked if we could hold the transfer temporarily because the trauma center was preparing to receive numerous trauma victims from a motor vehicle accident and that our patient being transferred was stable. I explained the request from the trauma center to the ED doctor and the patient and patient's family. The trauma center was going to call the ED back as soon as they would be able to handle any new transfers. We had to wait approximately fifteen to twenty minutes before we were given the word that it was time to transfer the patient. We did not want to place the patient on the long backboard, which was protocol for any patient going to the trauma center regardless of the injury prior to getting the go ahead for the transfer from the trauma center because the long backboards are very uncomfortable, and we did not want to cause any additional pain to the patient. The trauma center did call the ED in a timely fashion, and the transport took place, and a stretcher and staffs at the trauma center were available to take care of the patient without any further delays upon our arrival.

*****

We had a child that had special medical needs who would need to be transferred to the children's specialized hospital whenever she needed to be admitted as an in-patient. The first time my crew needed to transport the child, the mother asked if she could sit in the back of the ambulance with her daughter. The child needed frequent oral suctioning because of swallowing difficulties and the mother had her equipment with her in the ED. We placed the child on the stretcher and headed to the children's hospital. The mother asked if she could read her daughter a book during the transport, and I told her I would also love to hear a good story. She was reading her a story about princesses, and I commented that the three of us in the back of the ambulance were like the characters in the book. We arrived and went directly to the in-patient bed assigned. Many months later, we were dispatched to transport this same patient. Her mother was once again at her bedside armed with all the equipment and clothing needed for another in-patient admission. The mother once again asked me if she could ride in the back of the ambulance, and I said yes.

The mother said, "Thank you because the last nurse would not let me in the back with her."

My thought at that moment was why a nurse would separate a daughter and her mother, especially when the daughter had special needs. The daughter was the mother's entire world. The mother did everything for her daughter since the day she was born. The mother recognized me when I told her I hoped she had another book since I enjoyed the last story. I instructed my crew to move the patient's equipment and backpacks into the ambulance. Prior to the transport, the mother asked if we could change her. I had to find an adult diaper from the ED staff and assisted the mother while we changed her daughter and made her comfortable. We had extra pillows in the ambulance and used them to make her comfortable on the stretcher. We once again headed for the children's specialized hospital while the mother told me all about the accomplishments and things that her daughter loved to do.

*****

We were dispatched to transport a patient from an intensive care unit to another hospital for intervention for esophageal bleeding. When we arrived at the patient's bedside, he had a balloon-type device in his esophagus, attached to a trapeze with a weight on the end. I told the ICU nurse that we would not be able to maintain that setup in a moving ambulance. She had to call the attending doctor, and he said to disconnect the weights for the transport. My thought was if this patient begins to bleed, we might have to divert the transport to the nearest ED. His vital signs were stable and stayed that way during the transport, and he had no further bleeding. My way of approaching any task is that if you are prepared for the worst thing that can happen, then if something does change, you will be ready or, at least, have a plan to correct the change.

*****

The ED RN report I received was that there was an elderly dialysis patient with sepsis (an infection that has affected different body systems and organs) and was currently on a ventilator. We arrived to the ED and went to the room where the patient was. I looked at the cardiac monitor, and the cardiac tracing was normal, yet the blood pressure reading was very low, so I re-cycled the machine to take another blood pressure. The patient was unresponsive, yet that could be a result of either the low blood pressure or any medication given to the patient prior to our arrival. The reading was 70/46 just as the ED RN came back to the patient's bedside. I told the ED RN that she needed to contact the ED doctor and see if we can stabilize his blood pressure before he was transferred.

She said to me, "The doctor is off shift now."

And I explained to her to speak to the oncoming ED doctor since the patient was still in their care. I said that the patient was in septic shock based on his blood pressure and that the treatment for shock is intravenous fluids.

The ED RN responded, "He is a dialysis patient, so he can't have too many fluids."

The fear of fluid overload in a dialysis patient is very real, yet the patient must have a blood pressure high enough to send blood to the heart, lungs, and brain; and since he was already intubated and on ventilator, if he went into fluid overload, the patient would still receive oxygen. The ED RN returned with a bag of intravenous fluids and was going to connect it to an intra osseous (IO) site that had been started by the paramedics before the patient arrived to the ED. The site in the lower leg was already very swollen, and I advised the ED RN not to use that intravenous site since there would be no way of knowing if the fluids had infiltrated into the patient's leg. The patient had a triple lumen (three access ports) intravenous site in a large main vein, currently with two antibiotics running. The ED RN then went to connect the fluid intravenous to a small catheter in the patient's hand, yet the fluid would not run. The ED RN then took the IV tubing and hung it over the IV pole and walked out of the room. I looked at my EMTs and wondered what was going on. I connected the IV to the functioning triple lumen port and set it at the rate the doctor had ordered. The ED RN told the ED charge nurse that I was refusing to transport the patient, which was partly true based on his blood pressure.

The ED charge nurse came into the room, with his hand on his hip and asked, "Well, what blood pressure do you have to have before you can transfer the patient?"

I advised the ED charge nurse that I just wanted to see if IV fluids were going to elevate the patient's blood pressure. The patient's blood pressure did begin to come up, so we began getting our equipment ready and placing it on the patient. The ventilator was changed to our transport ventilator after we got the patient on our stretcher, and we were at this stage when the nursing supervisor came into the room and asked us how things were going. I explained that the patient's blood pressure was coming up, that he was already on our stretcher, and I was just getting one more blood pressure reading before switching the patient to the transport ventilator so we could leave. We switched the ventilator. He tolerated our ventilator well, and so we headed out, passing right in front of the charge nurse station, to our transfer destination. The patient did well during the transport, and when we arrived to the receiving hospital, the EMT in the back of the ambulance with me said to the patient, "Mr. Jones, we are here." The patient turned his head and opened his eyes and looked directly at the EMT. His blood pressure was now 90/72. When we got to the intensive care unit, I apologized for the delay, yet I explained the issue with the patient's blood pressure in the sending hospital.

The doctor then said to me, "I wondered why they were calling me for IV orders."

I had no idea the ED RN had called the receiving doctor for orders. All I could respond was "Well, at least the patient is more stable for you than he was for me."

*****

It was either Christmas Eve or New Years' Eve one year when we were dispatched to transport a forty-five-year old man to a hospital that provided invasive cardiac surgery. His diagnosis was a cardiac tamponade, which is when there is compression of the heart caused by fluid collecting in the sac surrounding the heart. We arrived shortly after being dispatched to find the patient agitated and very, very pale, and his blood pressure was extremely low. I questioned the ED nurse and doctor if there was any medication ordered to help raise his blood pressure. The doctor seemed anxious to get the patient moved from the ED and understandably so since the intervention needed was not available at this hospital.

The doctor said abruptly to me, "You cannot lay him down because of the cardiac tamponade."

I acknowledged that I was aware of this and asked the doctor for a medication to help raise his blood pressure. The doctor agreed, and the ED nurse prepared the medication so I could place it on the transport medication pump. The patient was restless and telling me that he was having severe back pain, so my crew and I loaded the patient on our stretcher and prepared for transport as fast as we could. The doctor advised the patient's family that the patient was critically ill at this point and that he may not survive the trip to the receiving hospital. As we were transporting, the patient's condition did not improve, and he became very diaphoretic (sweaty) and more restless. We increased the oxygen he was getting, and I called the receiving hospital's cardiac care unit RN to update her on the patient's status and what treatments were being given. When we arrived to the hospital, we went directly to the cardiac care unit and literally ran down the hall to the patient's assigned room. By the time we got our stretcher next to the hospital bed, the room was full of staff members including the cardiac care unit staff, the cardiac surgeons, and the respiratory therapist. The cardiac surgeon asked for a quick report, and I told him the status of the patient when we received him from the transferring hospital, the medication and treatments given during the transport, and his vital signs. I told the cardiac surgeon that the patient was demonstrating signs of AAA (Ascending Aortic Aneurysm) since he was restless, diaphoretic, complaining of severe back pain, and his abdomen was now distended and firm.

The cardiac surgeon yelled, "We are going to the OR now!" With that, the man was rushed down the hall to the operating room. I was in the cardiac care unit for approximately thirty minutes after the patient headed to the operating room so I could write my patient report since I had no time to write it during the transport. I never heard the outcome of the patient, yet the CCU nurse thanked me for calling with the updated report. She told me that she contacted the cardiac surgeon right after my phone call to her so he would be in the unit when we arrived, and the operating room would be prepared to accept the patient immediately.

*****

One night, the company dispatcher posted us in the City of Camden, which was a place we had not been posted for months. Each crew would position the ambulance in various response locations as per the dispatchers, throughout the shift. We received a dispatch for a seventeen-year-old male with a gunshot wound to the head in an ED, which is only 1.5 miles from a trauma center. We wondered why the patient had not been brought directly to the trauma center after the event. When we pulled up to the ED, we realized what had happened. There was a car near the ED's entrance, with yellow police caution tape around it, signifying that the patient was brought into the ED by a private vehicle. We went to the resuscitation room in the ED, and the staff was doing CPR on this young man, who was already intubated and had two or three intravenous lines. When the ED doctor wanted the staff to stop doing chest compressions to check for a pulse, I noticed that there was a gunshot wound to the boy's chest. I commented that my dispatch told me it was a gunshot wound to the head, and the ED doctor responded, "He has one there too." The staff was going to hang blood, so the hospital RNs did their double verification process per hospital protocol, and we put the bag on a pressure bag, which makes the fluid or blood run at a faster rate. There was no need to place the patient on our ventilator since it would take time to set up, and the trauma center was so close that we would continue to use the Ambu bag to ventilate the patient during the transport. The ED doctor confirmed pulses with a Doppler, so we quickly moved the patient, whose heart rate was in the thirties. Our protocol is to call the trauma center when we are fifteen minutes away, yet because of the short travel time, I was calling them as we literally ran out of the ED and told them we would be there in two to three minutes. My EMT driver put on the lights, used the siren, and we arrived in two minutes, yet during this time, the patient had lost pulses again, so I instructed the other EMT in the back of the ambulance with me to start chest compressions. We were still doing CPR when we arrived to the trauma center. After a short time, the extent of his injuries was too great, and he was pronounced dead. Everything from our end was as near to perfect as it gets. We were at the sending hospital from an area we are not usually posted in less than seven minutes. We were only in the ED for twelve minutes, and our transport time was only two minutes, yet his injuries were lethal. Days after this call, a day-shift EMT where I worked asked me if I was on this call, and I said, "Of course." He proceeded to tell me that one of his friends was working in the sending ED that night, and he said, "Your nurse did not waste any time. She just packed him up and went." Another EMT with whom I work with also asked me if I was on this call, and once again, I replied, "Of course." She told me that a friend of hers was working in the trauma center that night and had said, "Your nurse was calm and did all they could for that boy."

*****

We were leaving a hospital located in a rather bad side of town in Philadelphia one night when the ambulance driver slammed on the brakes and yelled, "Wow!" Since I was in the back of the ambulance facing the rear and I only have small windows in the back and side of the ambulance, I looked to up to see a person run directly behind the ambulance as the driver said, "He has a gun." Apparently, this man was running away with his head turned when he ran right into the side of the ambulance, bounced off, and kept on running while we got out of that area as quickly as possible.

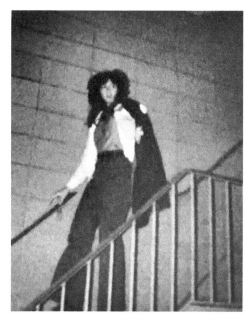

Susan on the volunteer first aid squad while going
to nursing and paramedic colleges

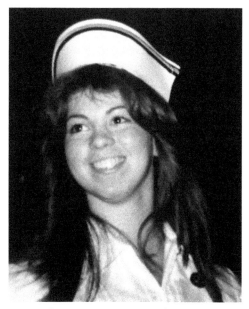

Susan at nursing graduation

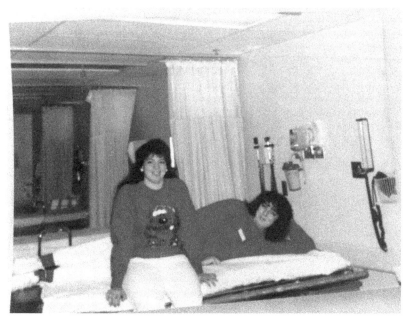

Susan and Debbie working Christmas In the ER in the 1980's

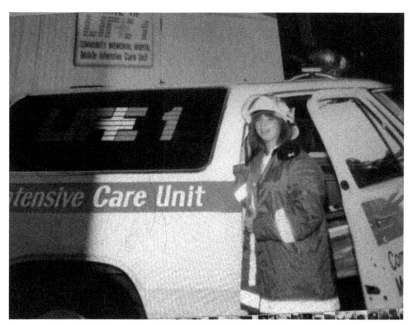

Susan as a Paramedic 1982

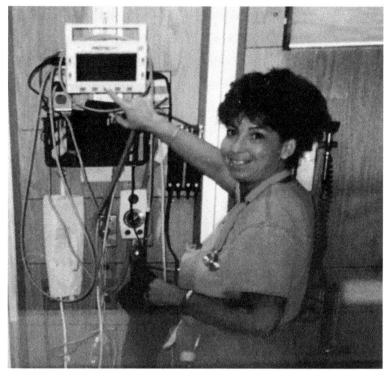

Susan as a nurse in ER

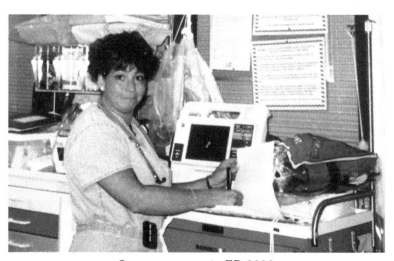

Susan as a nurse in ER 2000

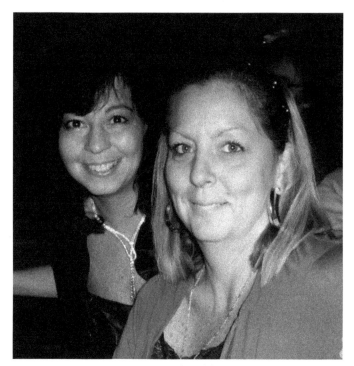

Susan and Debbie

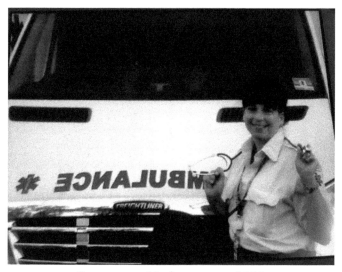

Susan as a critical care nurse 2015

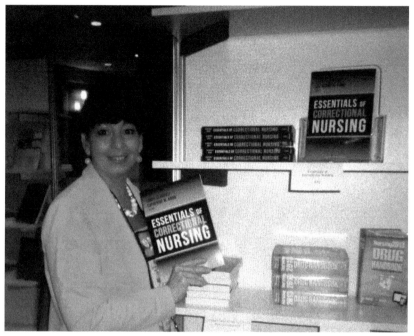

Release of textbook that Susan wrote a Chapter

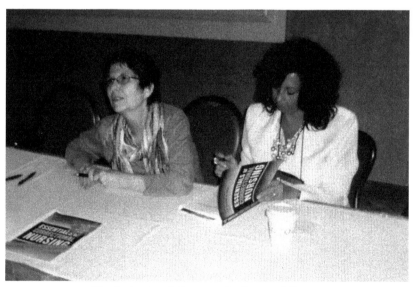

Book signing Margaret Collatt and Susan

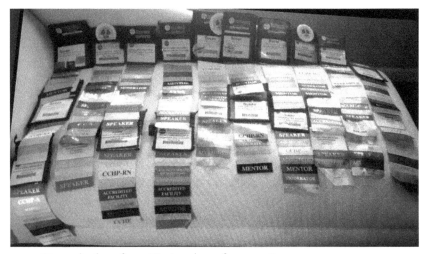

Name badges from National conferences Susan was a presentor

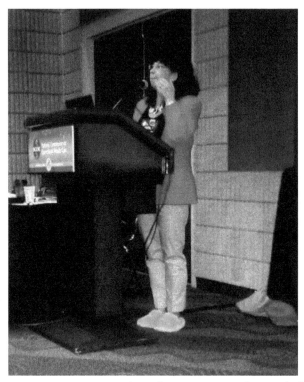

Susan presenting at a national conference wearing her pink slippers

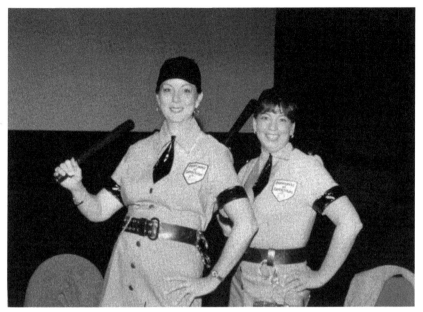

Susan and Debbie as correctional officers at a
Halloween party during a conference

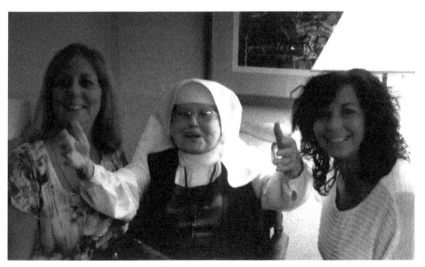

Susan and Debbie with Mother Antonia

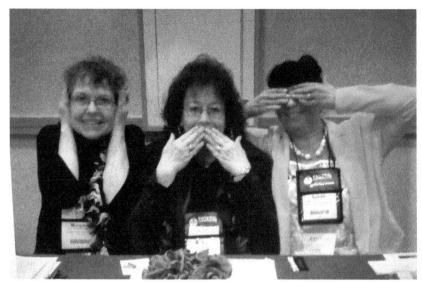

Margaret Collatt, Sue Medley Lane, and Susan having fun at a conference

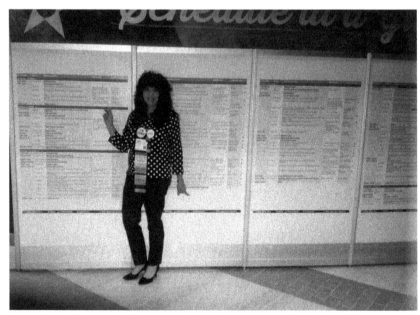

Susan pointing her sessions out on the schedule at a conference

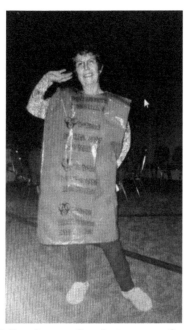

Margaret Collatt having fun during a conference session

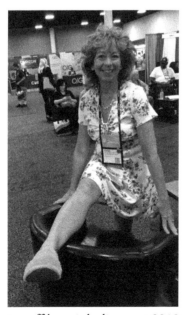

Susan showing off her pink slipper at 2019 conference

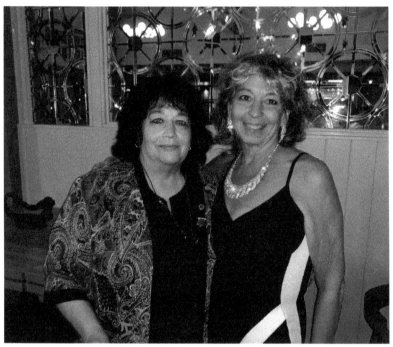

Sue Medly Lane and Susan at a dinner for people who have achieved the Certified Correctional Health Professional-Advanced status 2019

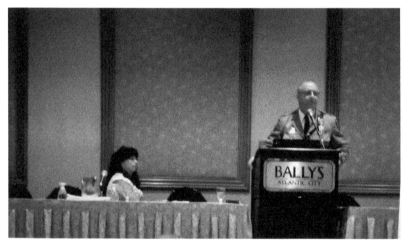

Susan and her husband Tom speaking about "active shooter" in hospitals at the NJ State Nurses Association conference

Nursing: Correctional Facilities

Once again, my best friend, Debbie, asked me if I wanted to work with her in a new place outside the emergency department. The only thing was that it was to be a nurse within the local county jail. I said I would go for an interview and was met at the main control entrance by the medical staff secretary who escorted me to the medical department. When we arrived to the medical unit, the secretary said to the administrator, "She did not jump when the doors slam like the girl yesterday." Over the years, I have worked in three different county jails in New Jersey with different titles such as staff nurse, director of nursing, and health service administrator. There are many names for those people housed in correctional facilities such as detainees, inmates, clients, yet for the medical staff, these people are simply called patients. The medical staff members are there to provide medical, dental, and mental health care to all patients in contrast to the correctional staff whose primary function is to provide a safe environment for all within the facility.

Not only are we providing these services, yet we are limited to the constraints of the correctional staff and rules of the facility. Upon entering the facility and heading toward the assigned medical unit, we had to go through many locked doors and a metal detector. We had to keep personal safety in the forefront of our minds at all times. Rules were in place to protect everyone—from devices that could be used as weapons such as syringes, needles, scalpels, and kitchen or maintenance equipment.

This facility had an *old jail* and a new building that had been built to house the county courthouse and the *new jail*. Both areas of the jail were in use, and they were connected by an underground tunnel between the two buildings. The dynamics of a correctional facility are a world of their own. There are correctional officers and administrative staff, medical staff, other civilian workers in the food industry, social service department, and the religious services to name a few. All correctional facilities are designed and set up differently, and the staffing is dependent on the number of people housed within

71

the facility. This facility housed approximately five hundred people, and we had both male and females in the facility. Our medical infirmary was located on the third floor of the old jail and was staffed by a nurse twenty-four hours a day, seven days a week. In this medical unit, we had cells in three different pods—one of which was for females, the other two for males—observation cells where the officer desk had windows to observe patients, and a protective custody cell that also had a sightline by the officer's area. The main housing units were on the fourth floor of the new complex with four main areas— North, East, West, and South—with smaller dorms being identified by letters *A, B, C,* and so on. There was an officer in each tower in each of the main four areas that controlled all the doors to that unit. The booking area, medical department, main control, visitation, and other administrative offices were on the third floor of this building.

The booking area was the area where people were brought to be processed into the facility, those being released from the facility, and those housed awaiting placement into a housing unit. We had patients that would be in the facility for anywhere from a few hours to a few years while awaiting trial. We had patients who liked to act out at times, mainly to break up the daily routine within the facility. One evening, Scott was acting out in the housing unit being loud, so he was brought down to the booking area to minimize problems in the housing area. He began to sing the song "Day-O" and kept doing so repeatedly. The booking officers told us to ignore Scott and not to encourage him in his singing as he was also yelling vulgarities to anyone walking past the cell. Toward the end of the evening, Debbie and I were heading to the elevators and walked by the booking cell Scott was in. We just had to stop in front of the cell, although the booking officers were telling us to just keep going, and join in with the sing-a-long, and the booking officers just shook their heads.

Scott later apologized to us for the things he yelled at us and said to us, "You know, I just had to put on a show."

*****

Another evening in the booking department, there was a young man in a booking cell who would not keep his uniform on and was flashing himself to everyone who walked by. Once again, the booking officers advised us to stay away from that cell and not to encourage his behavior. If you work in a correctional facility, you must have a tough skin and not take anything to heart. Once again, Debbie and I were working this evening and were back and forth in front of this booking cell numerous times during the evening. Toward the end of the evening, we went by the cell. The young man yelled at us, so, of course, we stopped. The young man must not have expected our reaction since after Debbie said jokingly, "Oh my goodness, it is so little." The young man turned around and put his uniform back on for the rest of the night.

*****

Sometimes people try whatever they can to get out of the facility, and the reason most people tried was that they had some kind of medical issue or condition that needed attention in the emergency department or in-patient hospitalization. I was working the night shift, and there was a man in one of the medical cells calling for a nurse. Accompanied by the officer in the unit, I went to the cell of the man calling. I honestly do not remember why he was being housed in the medical unit, yet he was standing at the cell door yelling, "You have to send me to the hospital!" When I asked him why I needed to send him to the hospital, he did not have a reason or a medical complaint, just continued to yell, "I want to get out of here. You have to send me to the hospital." After trying to get more information and attempting to take his vital signs, which he refused, he then looked at me as said, "Call me an ambulance."

I responded, "You're an ambulance." He then turned his back to me and went to lie on the bunk and did not say anything else the rest of the shift. Any nurse must trust their knowledge, experience, how the patient presents, and what is the patient's complaint to make a decision on any actions that need to be taken, yet in this environment, the nurse must be aware that the patient may simply be playing a con artist. If I ever had any doubt if any patient really needed to go to the hospital for an evaluation, then they were sent.

*****

Since this is a county jail and patients come in from the community, as opposed to being transferred to a state or federal prison from a county jail, one on the most challenging nursing issues comes from dealing with patients going through withdrawal from alcohol, drugs, or both. Seizures can be part of the withdrawal process, and the first seizure I had to deal with was only a few days into my employment at the jail. In fact, I was on my way to get my official facility identification badge; there was a call over the radio for a seizure in the visitation area. The middle-aged man was indeed having a grand mal seizure. The man denied alcohol use upon his screening into the jail, yet three days after being without alcohol, the seizure began right in the middle of a visit with his lawyer. He was sent to the hospital and admitted for alcohol withdrawal. When he returned to the jail, he was placed in the medical unit for a few days and did admit to drinking "a lot of vodka every day" for many years. Anytime he returned to the jail for another charge, he was automatically admitted to the medical unit for observation and treatment of alcohol withdrawal. The young woman who lived with him also was a regular at the jail and would also be admitted to the medical unit for alcohol withdrawal. She would go through the protocol of benzodiazepine administration, and on the fourth or fifth day of the medication, she would be clear of any withdrawal symptoms and never asked for medication after that point. They both later on in years died from illnesses related to chronic alcohol use.

In contrast, other patients thought that having a seizure meant an automatic transfer to the hospital. These patients get very creative, and some could win an Academy Award for their performance of having a seizure, yet they would always slip up just a bit to determine that the seizure was an act. One evening, I was working in the medical infirmary unit, and the officers called me for a person having a seizure. This patient was a new arrival to the medical unit on the day shift. I entered the cell with the officers to find the patient was on the floor, flailing his arms and legs around. As I observed the patient, his arm and leg movements stopped, and he opened his eyes and immediately said to me, "I just had a seizure, so I have to go to the hospital." This was the slipup I mentioned before. Patients who have had a true seizure do not awake to immediately speak clearly. Most patients are disoriented for a short period, and most do not remember the event. I evaluated the patient, took his vital signs, which were normal, and advised him to put his mattress on the floor so he would not fall off the bunk and strike his head. Shortly thereafter, the officers called me a gain for the same patient, once again having a seizure. After the event, he once again awoke immediately and said, "That makes two seizures, so you have to send me to the hospital now." I advised the patient that I would contact the medical director for any orders. I felt that this patient was trying to get out of jail way to hard, and asked the officers to call the booking desk and ask them what this patient's correctional charge was. I asked the officers if the patient had been on the telephone, and they were not sure, yet another patient in the medical unit told me that he had seen the patient on the phone right after dinner. The booking desk told us that this patient was a fugitive from Florida where he had a murder charge pending and that Florida officials were on their way to transfer the patient back to Florida for trial.

Debbie was working in the local emergency department, and later that evening, she called me and asked if I had a patient who was going to be sent to the emergency department for a seizure since she had "visitors" looking for the patient. I told her that my patient would not be going to the hospital. I advised the shift commander of the events that had happened and the call from Debbie. The correctional staff was on heightened alert until he was transferred the next day.

*****

Another patient came to the jail with a history of "seizures." As time went by, it was evident that this patient used his seizure history to obtain either attention from others or to get out of attending things like court appearances, going to work, and getting out of jail. I witnessed numerous episodes of this patient's seizures, yet once again, the patient did not exhibit typical symptoms after these episodes. We noticed that every time this patient was on the phone with his wife, he would have a seizure. His wife would call the jail over and over, saying that the medical department was not treating her husband's seizures, yet we were administering the same medication that the patient was on in the community. The patient was scheduled to go to court the next day, yet had another seizure the night before. He did go to court the next day, and his sentence was to report on a designated number of weekends to complete his jail time. Those people who came in to serve their terms on weekends would arrive to jail at 6:00 PM on Friday until 6:00 PM on Sunday evening. These people were appropriately called weekenders and were housed in cells on the first floor and did not mix with those serving time in the housing units unless they had to be placed in the medical infirmary.

One late Friday afternoon, I received a call from this "seizure" patient's wife who asked me to call the judge and advise him that her husband could not come to jail this weekend since the stress of coming to jail would cause him to have a seizure. I explained that I could not contact the judge, and if her husband did not come at his assigned time, then the court would put a warrant out for his arrest, and he would forfeit his weekend sentencing. The patient did come in as scheduled and did not have any more seizures.

*****

I was heading toward the jail to start my shift at 4:00 PM one day, yet there was a bomb threat in the courthouse in the justice complex, which is attached to the jail, so the road was blocked off by police, yet they waved me through knowing I worked at the jail. The sheriff department, local police department, along with the bomb squad was investigating a bag that was in one of the courtrooms. I received report from the day nurse who told me that one of the patients in the medical unit had a history of seizures, and the medication he is on is not a medication we carry in stock. The day nurse told me they called the prescription in to the local pharmacy, which was our backup pharmacy, but because of the bomb threat, they were not able to go to the pharmacy to pick up this medication.

The director of nursing said to me, "I will go get his medication in the morning."

I knew the patient had been without his medication for over twenty-four hours and did not want this patient to have a seizure. My friend Debbie was working on the ambulance in town that day, so I asked the officer in charge at the jail if Debbie (who also worked at the jail) could go get the medication from the pharmacy and bring it to the jail. He said he would have to clear it with the commander in charge of the bomb threat before he could say yes. He did make that call, and they said that yes, Debbie could bring the medication to the jail. I then had to call the pharmacy and advised them of the situation and explain that Debbie would be picking up the medication. During this time, the bomb threat was still going on, and we were told that the bomb squad was going to dismantle the device. Keep in mind that I could see the back of that courtroom through the window in the medical department. As Debbie and her partner came down the driveway, in the ambulance, the basement officer came over the radio asking if we had anyone going to the hospital since there was an ambulance coming down the driveway. I was there to get the medication from her, and I explained to the officer what was going on. I got the medication and a big cup of coffee from Debbie. The patient received his ordered dose, and the bomb was not a bomb after all. This patient did not have any seizures during his stay in the jail.

*****

One evening, I went in to the medical unit officer's control room where the two officers were talking, and I could not believe my eyes. There was a man standing in the window frame like Spiderman. I told the officers to look into cell B-1, and when they looked up, they could not believe it either. The window ledge was very narrow, and this was not a slim man, yet there he was. He was suffering from withdrawal symptoms and hallucinating when I went in to talk to him and check his vital signs. After we coaxed him from the window, I medicated him and continued to observe him the rest of the shift. The next evening, when I went to check his vital signs, he had no recollection of the events the evening before.

*****

Another evening, I was called to one of the medical cells for someone acting strange. When I got there, the man had his head in the toilet. I asked him to get away from the toilet, and when he did lift his head up, the water from his hair went all over the floor, and he almost fell down. This was a man who was over three hundred pounds, and he, too, was withdrawing from alcohol. We had to watch him one-on-one, so he would not injure himself and to make sure his condition did not worsen before he was sent to the hospital for evaluation and ended up being admitted to the hospital for alcohol withdrawal.

*****

It was a state law that we had to draw a blood sample to test each incarcerated person for syphilis. Since I worked most of my shifts in the medical infirmary, I would try to draw blood each evening on anyone who had been admitted into this unit. I had one person who came out of the medical dayroom and sat on the bench and said to me, "I don't like needles. Will you catch me if I faint?" When I told him that might be hard since I will have a needle in his arm. He was already pale and sweaty just with the thought of getting his blood drawn. He then asked me, "Are you good at this?" The officer said that I was the best at drawing blood, so he should just sit still. The patient then asked the officer if he would catch him if he fainted. At this point, I told the patient to sit on the floor and lean his back on the wall so if he did faint, he would not fall off the examination table. I told him to turn his head to the side, and I proceeded to draw his blood and was almost finished filling up the blood tube when he asked, "You will let me know when you're going to stick me, right?" The officer told him that I was almost done, and the patient then said, "That was not so bad." When the patient went back into the medical dorm, all the guys started laughing at him.

Another inmate came out for his blood test and said to me, "Ma'am, I don't do drugs anymore because I have no veins left."

I assured him that I would not stick him with a needle unless I felt I could get the blood draw on one try, and he agreed to that plan.

The officer said to the patient, "If she can't get it, no one will."

I did find a vein on the back of his forearm and obtained the specimen I needed. The patient thanked me for not "digging around looking for a vein" and went back into the medical dorm and said, "She is good!"

I had the same officers in the medical unit most of the time, and the running joke was they wanted to see how many blood draws I could do without missing, and they kept count each day. When I did one hundred blood draws without a miss, the one officer decided he would bring me a gift. He came in with a box of jelly doughnuts and said to me, "A bloody Mary would have been more appropriate, but I could not get that in here." When I hit two hundred blood draws without a miss, the other officer brought me an apple-shaped pin cushion. I kept this streak up, yet one evening, I had a patient literally jump off the examination table when I stuck him with the needle. The officer immediately got on the radio and announced, "She missed!"

*****

When our medical infirmary moved to a different location within the building, it had ten cells, most of which had two bunk beds, and one cell at the end of the hall had four bunks. We would house anyone withdrawing from alcohol or drugs, unstable mental health patients, suicide watch patients, patients on intravenous medication therapy, those on CPAP machines, and anyone else who needed to be isolated for an infectious disease. One evening, I arrived to nearly thirty patients in the medical infirmary, and in one cell, there were five people being housed. During the change of shift report, the registered nurse was told one of the patients had been having back and flank pain on and off all day. Motrin had been ordered by the doctor and administered, yet had no effect on the pain. I was working outside the medical infirmary taking care of the general population that shift. As the shift went on, his pain increased, and the other patients in that cell were yelling at the infirmary nurse to send him to the hospital. When I went into the medical infirmary to relieve the infirmary nurse for her dinner break, the patients in the cell started calling me to the cell to look at the patient. I assessed the patient, who at this time was restless, very uncomfortable, sweaty, and pale. He told me the pain was in his back and around to the front. I advised the patient and the others in the cell that the patient would be going to the hospital as soon as transportation could be arranged, and they seemed satisfied. The patient was sent to the hospital and diagnosed with a kidney stone. He received pain medication and a full evaluation at the hospital and was sent back to the jail later that evening. When the patient saw me after returning to the jail, he thanked me for taking care of him. The other nurse had taken care of him yet had not received any transfer orders from the doctors, so she felt her hands were tied. I explained to the health service administrator the next day that my concern was that if he did have a kidney stone and if that kidney stone blocked the ureter (the tube from the kidney to the bladder), then this patient's outcome could be detrimental to his well-being, so I re-called the physician for a transfer-to-the-hospital order.

*****

When I was working in the medical infirmary, we had a pregnant patient who was due to have her baby. She started having contractions on my shift, so I notified the health service administrator that there was a chance she would be sent to the hospital during the night. I knew that her contractions were not close enough or regular enough to send her out on my shift, so I asked the administrator if I could stay during the night shift to stay with the patient, so the other scheduled nurse could take care of the other patients in the medical infirmary that night. I explained to the patient that if she was sent to the hospital too early, they may examine her and return her to the jail to go further along in the labor process. She was comfortable with me staying with her that night and agreed she did not want to go back and forth between the hospital and the jail. As the night went on, her labor progressed, and she was doing well. She did go to the hospital early on the day shift and was admitted and later that day had a healthy baby, who was given to a family member as arranged by the social service department in the jail prior to the birth.

*****

When I was health service administrator at one county jail, the nurses were instructed to call me prior to calling the doctor or nurse practitioner on call for any medical emergency unless the emergency was life-threatening. One evening, I received a call from the registered nurse in charge who said that a female patient tried to hang herself in her cell. As the nurse was telling me about the incident, what treatments the staff had already done, and the patient's vital signs, I could hear yelling in the background only to find out that was the patient yelling. The nurse was calling me since she had called the doctor on call, and his orders were to put her on suicide watch, and he would see her in the morning. The reason for the call was because the nurse knew that this was not the most appropriate intervention for the patient. I asked the nurse if the patient had been placed in a cervical collar and placed on a long backboard to protect her cervical spine if there had been any injury, and she responded that yes, they had completed those tasks. I advised her to have the correctional staff call for an ambulance to have the patient evaluated in the local emergency department, which was also a trauma center. I notified the company regional manager the next morning to advise him of the events, even though it went against what the doctor had ordered the evening before. The regional manager asked me why I had approved the transfer to the hospital, and I told him that the patient could have internal injuries specifically to her spine and neck area that needed to be evaluated. I then told him that the patient had been admitted to the trauma intensive care unit with a diagnosis of carotid artery injury, and she would receive a mental health evaluation after she was medically cleared from her injury. The regional manager asked me how I knew that she had this injury, and I responded that I was a nurse and just knew the potential for this injury due to the mechanism of how she incurred the injury, and being a patient advocate, to agree with the nurses that evening that just placing the patient on suicide watch was not the appropriate treatment.

*****

One day, the deputy warden of this jail, who was in charge of the classification department, came to me regarding a patient who was writing to him daily to be transferred from this facility because he said he was not getting the proper diet for his diagnosis of diverticulitis. The classification department regulated all movement, housing units, and transfers for all those incarcerated at the jail. The deputy warden wanted me to look into it, so I reviewed the patient's medical file. The provider can order a medical diet, yet all diets in the facility are constructed and reviewed by dieticians on a frequent basis. I asked the officer in the medical unit to call the patient down so I could speak to him regarding the diet issue. I let the patient tell me about the food his medically ordered diet was comprised of and listened to his complaints.

Then the patient said, "When I was in Riker's Island, I had a different food." I advised him that different facilities may have different foods on medically ordered diets and that is the decision of the dietician, not the doctor or medical department. He started to get angry and once again started his sentence with "when I was in Riker's Island." Then I told him that we are in New Jersey, not Riker's Island, and there is no need to explain the same information over and over about his previous incarceration diets. I asked the patient to explain what diverticulitis was, and he said, "You're a nurse, don't you know?" I explained that I did know what this disease was, yet I wanted to make sure the patient had the correct information about the disease. After the patient told me that there were certain foods he could not have because it would aggravate his diverticulitis, I agreed that those foods could cause more discomfort or pain. I explained to the patient that if he wanted to refuse the diet that was ordered by the doctor, he would have to have a visit with the doctor to discuss the risks, and he could then sign a refusal of medical care specifically regarding the medical diet. He said he would think about it, so I asked the patient if he had ordered any food from the commissary during his stay, and he responded that he had. I told the patient that because of his medical diagnosis of diverticulitis, his commissary could be restricted to eliminate any foods that could cause him discomfort or pain. These were the foods he had described to me earlier in the conversation. He thought about it and told me that he would think about his options and get back to me. The patient left the medical department to return to his housing unit, and the medical officer said to me, "I didn't know you could restrict their commissary," and I responded, "I can't." About two weeks later, the deputy warden approached me to ask if the patient had been to state prison since he had not received any letters regarding his diet.

I said to the deputy warden, "We had a chat about his diet."

*****

The correctional facility had county, state, and federal standards, along with accreditation standards that had to be followed and maintained. One of the topics includes being prepared for emergencies within the facility. We would have disaster drills on a regular basis during all three shifts, and then the responses of correctional and medical staff would be reviewed and critiqued so policy and procedures could be updated or changed if needed. I spoke with the warden and the correctional officer in charge of training to propose a disaster drill to test the response and actions of the medical department staff as well as the interaction with correctional staff. I asked them if we could keep the scenario between just the three of us so no one in the facility would spread the word that this event was a going to be a drill, and they agreed. The scenario was that there was going to be an explosion in the kitchen resulting in various injuries after the dinner service was completed, which would be around 7:00 PM. I had to alter my hours that day because if I was in the facility that late, there would be suspicion that something was going on or about to happen. The injuries of those involved included a broken wrist, someone with chest pain, someone with back pain, someone with burns, and someone who had a massive head injury. I apologized to the warden because the person who was to have the fatal head injury was going to be the officer assigned in the kitchen, yet I wanted to demonstrate that the medical staff would assess the officer and realize there was no treatment for him and move on to evaluate the other patients who were all detainees. The warden, training officer, and I arrived to the kitchen and quickly explained the drill. We gave each person a paper that had their injury on it. Some of the patients were upset that they would not be getting back to their dorm to watch TV, yet when I explained that they were allowed to act out their assigned injury, they were happy to be involved, and they each did a great job. The call went over the radio as an explosion in the kitchen with heavy smoke, and the warden had already gone back to the main control room to advise the officer in charge that this was a drill, and no need to call the fire department or ambulance. The events unfolded as the training officer and I watched the actions of both the medical and correctional staffs independently and as they worked together. One of the standards stated that medical staff must respond to an emergency within four minutes. After about two minutes, the training officer said, "Where is the medical staff?" and I pointed to the other side of the kitchen where the medical staff members were standing because the kitchen had not been deemed safe yet by the correctional staff. As the last patient with the broken wrist was being escorted to the medical treatment area, there was another call over the radio that there was an officer down and a takeover of a dorm on the second floor. Keep in mind that the officers that responded to the kitchen had to put on breathing apparatus and protective equipment for the medical disaster drill and now had to get out of that equipment and into riot-type gear. As I was walking down the main corridor back to the medical department when the takeover call came over the radio, I looked up to the main control room to see the warden smiling. He decided to piggyback his disaster, which only he knew about, onto the scenario I had developed. As the officers arrived up to the second floor, they realized it had been a drill. The warden wanted to have a short meeting after these "disasters" with the training officer and me to get our perspective on how the medical and correctional staff responded.

At the end of this meeting, I simply said to the warden, "I will not invite you to anymore of my disaster drills!" and we all laughed. When we discussed these drills with other administrative staff a few days later, it was decided that both the medical and correctional staff did a great job, and that no policies or procedures needed to be changed.

*****

We had a patient who wanted to get out of jail, so he drank cleaning fluid from a cleaning bottle in the dormitory area. He was brought to the medical unit for evaluation, and poison control was contacted. The cleaning fluids are nontoxic and diluted with water before the bottles go into the dorm specifically for this reason, so the amount of cleaner was so minimal that poison control just recommended that we observe the patient. I had to go to the warden's office to report our findings, report poison control recommendations, and advise the warden that the patient did not have to be sent to the hospital for evaluation and that the patient was placed in a cell in the medical department for observation. When I told the warden that the patient should not experience any side effects and that he was now going to be clean inside and out, all he could do was laugh.

*****

I received a call on a Monday, which happened to be Labor Day, from a nurse in the medical department advising me that there had been a patient death. I was supposed to be off that day, yet I headed to the jail, which was one hour away. When I got there, the deputy warden said, "You can't help him now. Why did you even come in?" I advised him that I felt I needed to be there in case any of the nurses needed my help. The nurse that morning was administering medication from dorm to dorm, and when they arrived to the patient's dorm, he did not come to the door for his medication, so the officer went into his cell and found him on his bunk. The patient was being treated with medication for mental health issues. The nurse was also the nurse who administered evening medication the night before, so she was visibly upset, and so I had another nurse complete the medication run.

Word of the patient's death spread through the jail like wildfire, and investigators had to be called in. There would have to be an investigation called a mortality review from the medical department as well as an investigation by the county representatives. The next day, in the daily warden's morning briefing, the warden advised us that the time of death had been determined to be approximately 1:00 AM. There would be an autopsy to determine the actual cause of death, yet it appeared to be an overdose. The warden asked me, "What medication did he overdose on?" and I responded that we would have to wait for the drug screen to determine that since it may not have even been any of the medication the patient was prescribed that caused his death.

One of the primary functions of the nurses administering medication is to make sure that the patients actually swallow any medication that is administered since patients occasionally hoard their medication and sell or trade them with other patients for other things such as food or drugs. My concern was that the warden would blame the medical department for the patient's death since it appeared to be an overdose, yet he was more upset with the correctional staff because of the estimated time of death of 1:00 AM. His concern was that officers were to check patients on scheduled rounds on all shifts to verify all those incarcerated in the jail were living and breathing.

*****

I was working as the director of nursing at a county jail and working the night shift one night to cover the registered nurse who was off on vacation, and there was a terrible thunder and lightning storm. I walked into the medical unit to find over twenty detainees who needed to have their initial medical screening, which included vital signs, weight and height, medical and psychological screening, and patient consent for treatment, and administration of a tuberculosis test. I was working with a licensed practical nurse, and we just started a production line, and in about two hours, all the detainees were screened and assigned to housing units.

*****

Another day, when I was just about to leave for the day, I heard on the radio a call for a person having a seizure in the female housing unit. This detainee had been in the hospital for cardiac issues a few days earlier yet signed herself out against medical advice because she had told one nurse that the nurses in the jail took better care of her than the nurscs in the hospital. When the medical staff arrived to the female housing unit, it was determined that the woman was in cardiac arrest, so CPR was initiated. Emergency response was called, and she was brought to the medical department. We continued to do CPR until the paramedics arrived, and she was transported to the hospital where she later died.

*****

There was a young man who had a fainting episode in one of the main housing units, so he was brought to the medical department for observation since he had no medical problems yet was on medication for depression. The next morning, he had another episode, so he was sent to the hospital for evaluation and admitted with an elevated blood sugar. He was diagnosed with new onset diabetes and sent back to the facility after his hospitalization. The nurses had to teach him how to draw up and give himself insulin in the days after his return. The day that he was sent to the hospital, his commissary order came in, and it was full of candy. We came to find out that he was not eating the meals served by the facility and just eating candy.

*****

We had a patient in the medical department who had been diagnosed with cancer and was failing. He had no family and no place to go if he was released from jail, and he told staff members that he did not want to go anywhere else to die because he felt he knew the staff within the facility. It was a Friday evening, and I received a call from the nurse on duty, and she said that his vitals, level of consciousness, and respirations were changing, and she asked if she could stay with him through the night so he would not die alone if that time came. He had signed the Do Not Resuscitate consent, and the security staff was made aware of the plan that was the wishes of the patient. The day shift was informed in a report what the plan was, yet around 9:00 AM, I received another call that the day nurse had sent him to the hospital because he was dying. I was upset with this nurse's actions since it went against everything that had been planned, and most importantly, it went against the wishes of the patient.

Nursing: Cardiac Care Unit (CCU)

There was an older lady who weighed about 110 pounds admitted to the CCU. She kept having runs of ventricular tachycardia (V-tach), which can be life-threatening if not corrected. She would call the nurses and say, "It is happening again." Some episodes would resolve without intervention, and a few times, we had to shock her. She was on a drug called lidocaine to reduce these irregular heartbeats, yet a few hours into the shift, we noticed that she was picking at things in the air and becoming confused, which is a sign of becoming toxic to the medication. I do not even remember how many times we called the admitting physician, yet at one point, I suggested a newer drug we were using as paramedics called bretylium, which treated the same irregular heartbeats. He agreed to start that medication and discontinue the lidocaine, and that lessened the irregular heartbeats, and the patient remained coherent. When the physician came in around 6:00 AM to see the patient, she again went into V-tach. After the episode, the physician said to us, "I cannot believe she just went into that rhythm right in front of me." All we could do was shake our heads and think that now the physician knows how we felt all night.

*****

One night, we were expected to get severe thunderstorms. Our hospital was on a canal, and all the rooms in the CCU had big windows overlooking the water. The lightning show was impressive, yet for some reason, I had a bad feeling. We had four patients on ventilators that night, but there were only three nurses. My thought was what if the power goes out? The other nurses were not concerned because they said we have backup generators that will turn on. We double-checked to make sure all the ventilators were plugged in to the emergency outlets that were connected to the power source from the generators. I still had that feeling, so I went to the step-down unit, which we shared a break room with and explained our situation. We agreed that a nurse from the step-down unit would come over immediately if we lose power. We all had flashlights in our pockets and were ready just in case. We all knew which room we were going to if needed. Honestly, it was not fifteen minutes later that the sky lit up, and then thunder boomed so loud that it shook the building, and off went the power. We all ran to our designated rooms, including the step-down unit nurse. The generator did turn on, yet it was about a forty-five-second delay. All the patients were all right. The respiratory therapist came charging into the unit once the generators were on and did not know where to go first. We told him what we had done, and he breathed a sigh of relief. Once the event was over, one of the other CCU nurses looked at me and asked me, "How did you know that was going to happen?" I explained that I did not know, but I wanted to be prepared if it did occur.

*****

"Code Blue CCU, Code Blue CCU!" the hospital operator said over the hospital intercom.

They always state the message in that format, but this time, we really had two cardiac arrests happening at the same time. As the respiratory therapist, the house doctor, and the nursing supervisor arrived, they all asked, "Which room?"

Our answer was room 3 and room 6! We got the help we needed, and both patients survived.

*****

While working full-time, three nights per week in this CCU, I was also working full-time, three nights per week as a paramedic. One night, I went in to see my patient Mrs. Smith after the change of shift report. She was admitted the night before with unstable angina. I introduced myself and asked Mrs. Smith how she was feeling.

She said, "Good now. I had chest pain last night, and those paramedics came and brought me to the hospital."

I said to her, "They gave you nitroglycerin, and you felt better. And you did not even want to come to the hospital."

She looked at me, and she might have been thinking that I must have gotten a really good report from the previous nurse to know all that. I then asked her if I looked familiar and went on to explain that I was the paramedic in the ambulance with her the night before. We both laughed, and then she thanked me for taking away her chest pain.

Paramedic: Mobile Intensive Care Unit

I worked on Life 1, which was the first and only paramedic unit in Ocean County, New Jersey, at that time, and there were over fifty retirement villages within that county. I started as a full-time night-shift paramedic from 7:00 PM to 7:00 AM. We were based out of a local first aid squad initially until the hospital built a more permanent building for us. The first aid squad members of that building were very kind and welcoming. Some would bring us freshly baked cookies and food since at that time, there was only one place to get food until 8:00 PM. They liked to have us show them and explain to them what equipment we had and what we could provide to patients. Paramedics were a new concept in New Jersey at that time. Not only was the concept of pre-hospital care new, the fact that there were females in this profession was also new. When they ordered our uniforms, I had to get small or extra-small uniforms and coats since there were none being made for women at that time.

Our initial coverage area was a group of towns near where we were based. Our trucks and equipment were brand-new, and the eight full-timers were ready to save the world. Yet we had to face the fact that many of the volunteer first aid squads thought of us as taking over when, in reality, we were there to provide advanced medical care to their patients. We were canceled by the first aid squads while en route to the call many times. We had to do a lot of public relation work to make them feel comfortable with this new concept of treating patients in the field since our vehicle did not have the capability to transport patients. We had two drug boxes that we alternated on odd and even days to keep the stock in use, an airway box, an EKG monitor, a trauma bag, and a radio to talk to medical control at the hospital.

I was in the back of an ambulance once getting ready to start an intravenous on a patient, and a volunteer stated, right in front of the patient, "I was a nurse, and you cannot use that needle without sterilizing it first." I explained to her and the patient that the needles and syringes we carry are already sterilized and only for single use and proceeded to start the intravenous line.

Another barrier we had to overcome was the fact that doctors were not used to this type of pre-hospital treatment. Imagine, if you will, the doctors being told to give paramedics medical orders for patient care when the doctor did not even see the patient. In the beginning, most doctors would give us "monitor and transport the patient" orders even when we had the capability to provide medication that could improve the patient's condition. Once, we had a patient involved in a car-versus-tree accident, and he was trapped in the car. While the fire department worked on extricating the young man from the vehicle, our orders from the doctor at the hospital were "Get him here now!" We worked through this with time after the doctors understood what medications and procedures we could do in the field and after they knew us better and trusted the patient reports we were providing.

*****

My first call as a paramedic was a patient with chest pain whom we gave nitroglycerine to, and the patient's pain went away. I felt as though we were doing the right thing and helping people in medical need before they got to the hospital.

The second call I had as a paramedic was an infant in cardiac arrest. The call was confusing because the dispatcher stated, "We don't know if the infant is not breathing or bleeding" because the caller was frantic on the phone (pre-911 emergency call system). We arrived, and police cars were all over the street and lawn, and we went to the downstairs of a split level-home, and the first aid members were doing CPR on an infant. They did not know what we could do, nor did they know what equipment we carried, so we told them to continue CPR and move to the ambulance. We were told on the way out of the house by a family member that the infant had a congenital heart defect that could not be corrected with surgery. If anyone has taken a CPR class, this child looked like the infant they have you train on. We continued to do CPR and provide care until our arrival at the emergency department. The child was pronounced dead a short time later. Then I began to question my decision to be a paramedic. I told myself that we did the best we could do, yet it was their time to go.

*****

I was driving the paramedic unit, and we were at a red light at a very busy intersection with about four cars in front of me. As we were talking, all of a sudden, I heard the sound of crashing metal and breaking glass. We both looked around and saw that a tractor trailer had made a right-hand turn from the left lane, to clear the corner where light poles, electrical wires, and lighted sign were about ten feet from the curb. Then I saw a small car crushed under the truck, yet the truck was attempting to continue the turn not knowing that it was a car under his truck and not the curb that was holding him back. We turned on all the lights and sirens, yet because of traffic, we could not move. I ran to the car, and my partner ran to the truck driver to tell him to stop moving. I was not sure what I would find when I got under that truck since the roof of the car had been collapsed down to the hood level. I was able to see inside the door, which had popped open when the force hit the roof of the car, and a man said, "I think I am okay." This man had the quick thinking to release the seat back when he saw the truck wheel heading toward his car, so he was lying flat in his driver's seat with the roof of his car only inches from his body. The fire department came and extricated the man from the car, who only had some minor scratches because of broken glass that had hit him.

*****

As most people know, there is a joke when talking to people from New Jersey by saying, "What exit?" as related to the two main north and south highways—the New Jersey Turnpike and the Garden State Parkway. The exits represent mile markers with the lowest numbers being in south Jersey, and the numbers go up as you go north on each of these highways.

On another night shift, when I was driving, we were dispatched to a chest pain call that was about fifteen miles from the hospital. We got on the Garden State Parkway and headed south. Traffic was heavy yet moving, and people were yielding to us in the fast lane. I looked in my review mirror and saw a New Jersey State Trooper coming up behind me with his lights on. I could not move into the slow lane at that point because all the other people had moved over into that lane for us. As we were approaching a rest area that had the exit to the left, we got canceled from the call by the dispatchers via the radio. I turned off the lights and exited into the rest area so we could head back north to our base area. With that, the State Trooper followed us still with lights on, so I pulled over to let him go by. But he did not go by. Instead, he pulled behind us and exited the vehicle walking up toward our truck. As he approached the driver's window, he said, "License and registration." He had a bewildered look on his face. I was not sure if he was surprised that a female was driving the truck and had no idea what his issue was at the time. While holding the credentials in his hand, he asked, "Why did you have your lights on?" I told him that we were on our way to a chest pain call yet just got canceled by the county dispatchers. His response was "Who can verify that you got canceled from that call?" I advised the State Trooper that the county dispatcher could verify any information about this call. After a few minutes, he gave back the credentials and walked away.

I said to my partner, "What was that all about?"

A few days later, when I was telling another paramedic the story, he shed some light on why the State Trooper may have pulled us over. The other paramedic told me that the night before our encounter, he was driving on the same road going to a call, and there was a State Trooper in the lane in front of him, no lights on doing the speed limit. The paramedics were responding to a cardiac arrest, so they tapped the air horn a few times, yet the State Trooper would not speed up or move over. This went on for miles. The paramedic crew called the county dispatchers and asked them to contact the State Police dispatcher and advise this State Trooper to let the paramedic unit pass. We speculated that the State Trooper who would not let the paramedic unit pass was the same State Trooper that pulled us over. We think he thought that it would be the same crew as the night before, and he was going to question them why they called Trooper dispatch. That explains the bewildered look the State Trooper had when he approached our truck and found a female was driving, and he knew then that it was not the same crew since the crew the night before were two males.

*****

If you provide medical care for any length of time, you will witness different treatment modalities, different medications, different medication dosages and indications for use, different equipment, and different duration of how long all these medical provisions are around depending on research and evaluation. One such treatment modality was the use of medical anti-shock trousers (MAST), which had three sections that could be inflated with air using a manual foot pump to apply pressure to the lower extremities and abdomen and pelvis region to shift the patient's blood volume up to the vital organs such as the brain, heart, and lungs. You would lay the MAST pants out flat and place the patient on top of it using Velcro to wrap each leg and the abdominal section. Then you would have to connect the foot pump to each section and pump up that section. If this treatment was used in the pre-hospital setting, they were never removed prior to arriving at the hospital since removing them quickly could mean that the patient would lose their blood pressure or begin to hemorrhage or both, so there was a sign sewn into them that said "Do Not Cut." We did use this treatment modality a few times, and once, when we used them on a trauma victim and arrived at the hospital, we heard the doctor say, "I don't believe in these," and proceeded to rip the Velcro open. The patient went into cardiac arrest and died a few minutes later.

Another old treatment modality that we tried was called rotating tourniquets. This was used for people in congestive heart failure (originally called pulmonary edema). We would put tourniquets on three extremities and manually rotate them every fifteen minutes, which was not too bad for paramedics since their time spent with the patient is usually short. Yet once this modality was started, it had to be continued or weaned off by the emergency department nurses, which could be very time-consuming depending on the patient's response to medication or dialysis to remove the fluid. This, too, is no longer a treatment modality since the evolution of medications and ventilator support such as BiPAP.

*****

We were treating an elderly female who had a complaint of chest pain and had treated her with nitroglycerine, and she became pain free and had stable vital signs. When we were a few minutes from the hospital, the medical control doctor, via the radio, gave me an order for atropine 0.5mg IV. I wondered why she was giving me that order since the patient's heart rate was at a regular rhythm of six-ty-two beats per minute. Atropine is a medication given to increase the heart rate thereby providing oxygenated blood to vital organs such as the heart, lungs, and brain. I questioned the doctor about the order, and she responded, "Give the atropine now! Their heart rate is thirty!" I looked at my monitor, and it said sixty-one. I palpated the patient's radial pulse and listened to her heartbeat, and both were six-ty-one beats per minute. I recorded EKG strips for documentation. I told the doctor I was not giving that atropine and that we were less than a minute away from the hospital. I knew this doctor was going to ream me out, yet it was not indicated. We got to the emergency department and connected the patient to the cardiac monitor. The patient's heart rate was still in the sixties. Her blood pressure was within normal range. Her color was pink. The skin was warm and dry, and she was free of chest pain. The doctor, after checking on the patient, came at me as expected with an EKG tracing in her hand. She shouted, "Why did you disobey my order? The patient's heart rate was thirty," as she handed me the EKG tracing. While explain-ing my reasoning, I noticed that her EKG tracing looked different from mine and realized that the speed button on the recorder was pushed so that the paper was actually moving faster while printing, thereby making the heartbeats being spread out. As I pointed this out, the physician simply walked away. She never did thank me or apologize to me for yelling at me over the radio or in the emergency department.

*****

We got a call for a car-versus-tree accident one early morning around 5:30 AM. The hospital where we were based was at Exit 82, and this call was for mile marker 58. We headed south, with no traf-fic in sight since it was early and a Saturday. When we arrived, the State Trooper car was in the shoulder of the road. This area is known as the Pine Barrens, so there are a lot of pine trees lining the parkway.

We got out of our truck, gathered all our equipment, and headed toward the Trooper. He pointed to a ragtop-covered jeep that had impaled itself into a tree. The problem was that there was a drainage ditch between the road and the tree, so it was actually suspended into the tree about five feet up from the ground. My partner, who is a foot taller than me, got up into the jeep to find the patient lying across the back seat of the jeep unresponsive. As I handed all our equipment up to him, I asked the Trooper to please give me a boost so I could get up there and help. He took a moment but then helped me. At this time, the fire department and volunteer ambulance squad arrived, and we had to get this young man in critical condition out of the back seat of the jeep onto a long backboard to lower him to the ground, all without putting too much weight on the impaled jeep. At this time, in pre-hospital treatment, you had to take patients to the closest hospital for care. The only trauma center in New Jersey at that time was over one hundred miles away, and there was no such thing as medical flight teams. The young man was alive, with a flail chest (where there are numerous fractured ribs), a punctured lung, and internal bleeding that we knew of. I later found out that he died as result of the injuries he sustained.

*****

On a different call on the Garden State Parkway, we headed north from Exit 82 to Exit 96.8 southbound for a vehicle-versus-tree case. As we approached going north, we had to find a place to cut over to the southbound lanes. The Garden State Parkway only has a few turnaround points for emergency vehicles even though the freeway is 172 miles long. In this portion of the road, there are trees in the median, and most areas have drainage areas off the shoulder that can dip down a few feet. As we were coming up to the mile marker on the northbound side, we were advised to expedite our response since the patient was bleeding out. We crossed over the median over some really rough terrain, and I was not driving this time. The fire department had already removed the passenger side door and was working on the driver side door as we approached. In the driver's seat was a young man that was extremely pale and had blood coming from his nose and mouth. My partner was clearing large clots out of the patient's mouth when the driver side door came off. I stood on the door and connected him to the cardiac monitor, and he had a pulse of about twenty. Honestly, I was surprised he even had a heart rate with the condition he looked. I began the task of starting intravenous lines while trying to get into this mangled car that had wrapped around the tree. When we went to move the patient onto the long backboard to get him out of the car, we saw massive amounts of blood under him on the seat and saw that his pelvis was wide open. He coded in the ambulance, and we continued CPR and advanced life support until we got to the hospital, yet he succumbed to his massive injuries. It would later be determined that this young man was from North Jersey heading to the Jersey Shore on a Friday night after working until the early hours of the morning and most likely fell asleep at the wheel since there were no skid marks noted on the road and the curvature of the road would lead right into that tree. For many years, I saw that same battered tree at mile marker 96.8 and thought of that young man. Eventually that tree was removed for road expansion, yet I will never forget that spot or that young man.

*****

We had just started our shift, and it was a summer night about 8:00 PM when we got dispatched to a motorcycle-versus-tree case. We arrived fairly quickly and found the patient against the tree, and the motorcycle was about twenty yards away lying in the grass. At the base of this tree was a big bush with thorns on it. After we got the patient away from the tree and bush, it was evident he needed to be intubated and was in shock. While I was preparing to start the intravenous lines, my partner began the task of intubation while lying in the grass. I looked up as we were working on this young man and saw a middle-aged woman running right toward us. A police officer stopped her, and we continued working on the patient while she screamed, "My son, my son! God, help him!" He was still alive yet had massive internal injuries, evident from the large bruises on his chest and abdomen, how dangerously low the vital signs were, and that he was unresponsive. We loaded the patient into the ambulance and headed to the hospital, which was about four minutes away. While en route to the hospital, we needed to go through one of the most congested intersections in the town, so we had a police escort. There was a police officer in front of the ambulance, our medic unit driven by a fireman behind the ambulance, and another police car behind that. In the ambulance were the driver, my partner and I working on the patient, an EMT doing cardiac compressions, and another EMT providing ventilations via the intubation tube. We were about half-way to the hospital, coming up to that busy intersection, when the driver yelled, "HOLD ON," and the ambulance screeched to an abrupt stop. All of us in the back of the ambulance except for the patient were tossed around. I ended up thrown into the side door steps, and the medication box, which was open, flew off the bench and fell on top of me. We all got back to the task at hand and headed for the hospital once again. We later found out that a woman tried to make an illegal left turn at that intersection between the lead police car and the ambulance. The young man never regained pulses and died in the emergency room. For all the years I lived in that town after this tragic event, the bark on the tree that he hit had never recovered.

*****

We were dispatched to a gunshot wound to the head and arrived on the scene, which already had numerous police vehicles present. The officer said that the patient was inside, yet that I could not go in. When I asked him why, he said something like, "It is a mess in there." My partner remembers me being really "hot" over that. I did not go in, yet my partner later told me that there was a small older woman with a gunshot wound to her head with her arms folded across her chest and a shotgun next to her. The patient was pronounced dead at the scene by the medical examiner.

*****

Weather in New Jersey can be tough at times. It can be unbearably hot and humid, freezing cold, rain for days causing flooding, hurricane-like storms, and crazy snowstorms. It had been snowing all day, and we made our way into work for the 7:00 PM–7:00 AM shift. We were based at the hospital, and the emergency department was very empty. We got a call for a "sick person" in a retirement village that would normally take about ten minutes to get to. It took us close to forty-five minutes to get there, through the falling snow, howling winds, and lightning. It was really crazy out there, and as we turned the corner to the street the call was on, a bolt of lightning came down, hit a telephone pole, and the whole left side of the street went dark. I remember saying to my partner, "In North Jersey, we either have snow or lightning, not both at the same time!" The call we were going to was on the side of the street that still had power. The ambulance was already there, and we got into the house, and there was a suitcase at the door and a person with a winter coat, gloves, and boots on standing inside the door. When we asked where the patient was, the man by the door said, "I am. I just wanted to go get checked out at the hospital." He had no particular complaint. So he was assisted to the ambulance. While driving back out of the retirement village, we were behind the ambulance. All of a sudden, they were heading toward the right. My guess is they were following the street lights since visibility was really poor, yet they were heading toward a light on a house porch. We had to call the county dispatcher to advise them that they are not on the road anymore. Luckily, we did not have any more calls in the snow that shift.

*****

Being the only paramedic unit in the county caused some questions at times. During another blizzard, we received a phone call from the county dispatchers. They asked if we could respond to Ocean Gate. I had to ask my partner since I did not even know where Ocean Gate was. It was about thirty minutes away, on a normal day. They said they had a burn victim they wanted us to respond to. As we headed past the hospital to go south to Ocean Gate, keeping in mind we have already been on the road close to forty-five minutes by now, the dispatchers contacted us and said, "The patient is refusing treatment, but the police want you to continue to respond." During the trip south, I had intravenous bags of lactated Ringer's in my jacket to warm them up. We did have a heater in the truck, yet it was so cold outside they were still cold. We finally got to the town of Ocean Gate, and the police officer told us to follow him to the patient's house. When I got out of our truck, the snow was midway to my thighs. We got into the house to find police officers and first aiders around the patient. She was lying on the bed, with burned hair, no eyebrows, and had burns to her neck, face, chest, and arms. She was awake, not aware of the events that had happened, rambling and refusing to go to the hospital. There was a strong odor of alcohol present. I asked the patient her name and if she had been drinking any alcohol. She said that she had been drinking all day because of the snow and asked me why everyone was in her house. I explained to her that she had burns and needed to go to the hospital now. She finally said okay, and we wrapped her in the bed sheets that had an outline of serous fluid all around her body, then wrapped the sheets and the patient in burn sheets. The doctor wanted us to start an intravenous to provide fluids that had been lost. The traditional areas of hands, arms, and neck were all burned to varying degrees. I asked a police officer to hold the IV bag up high for me while I started an intravenous in the ankle, and it ran like a charm. We had to slide her across the snow on a Reeves stretcher to get her to the ambulance. We covered her in blankets and turned up the heat in the ambulance. I was so hot I took my coat, sweater, and scarf off for the ride. It took us almost an hour to get to the hospital. When we went to move the patient over to the hospital stretcher, I had to warn the nurses to hang the IV bag at the foot of the bed since her IV was in her ankle.

The ER doctor made a comment. "Wow, fancy."

I told him I did not have much of a choice as he would quickly find out when the blankets were removed. She got moved to a burn center where she later died of an infection.

During one of these snowstorms, I guess the day-shift paramedics had some free time on their hands because when I got to work that night, there was a tall snowman spray-painted to look like a paramedic outside in the yard where the paramedic unit was based.

*****

One spring evening, we had literally just got on duty when we got a call for a sixteen-year-old male electrocuted behind an apartment complex. In normal driving time, it would take approximately twenty minutes to get from our location to the call location, yet we got there in approximately eleven minutes. We had a paramedic student riding with us that shift. We got to the apartment complex parking lot and have to carry all our equipment down this embankment to where the patient was. Above us were massive power lines. We had not worked with members of this first aid squad before since it was not in our designated response area. They were doing CPR, and we began the tasks of advanced medical treatments such as intubation, starting intravenous lines, and defibrillation when appropriate. We defibrillated the young man once and did get a heart rhythm back, yet he went back into the lethal ventricular fibrillation rhythm again. We were giving all the advanced cardiac life support drugs as they continued CPR. Before we attempted to move him back up this embankment to get him to the ambulance, a police officer told us that his father was "up on the hill with chest pain." I looked up the hill, and there were about fifty to seventy-five people up there looking down on what we were doing. I advised them to take the father to the hospital immediately and that we would be transporting very soon. We had to carry the patient up the hill on a Reeves stretcher while coordinating CPR and ventilations. Once loaded in the ambulance, it only took about forty-five seconds to get to the hospital. They continued to provide medical care and CPR on this young man yet to no avail. The power line he had come in contact contained some massive voltage going through it, so the result was not surprising, yet we tried our best. During this whole event, the paramedic student just watched while we did what we had to do. Unfortunately, sometimes you just do not have the time to explain each task you are performing when time is truly of the essence, so we talked about what we did, why we did each task, and the challenges we faced later that evening with the student.

*****

On the Fourth of July, one seaside town would put on a firework display over the beach. We got dispatched to a person struck by a firework shell. As we approached the scene, there were a mass number of people condensed in the area we needed to get to. The patient was an approximately eight-year-old boy who was there with his mother watching the fireworks when an undetonated firework shell came down from the sky and struck the young boy in the head. The first aid squad had already bandaged his head yet the dressing was soaking wet with blood, and the boy was unresponsive. My partner and I got in the ambulance and began to intubate him and start intravenous lines. At the side door to the ambulance was a man yelling at us to get the boy to the urgent-care facility down the street. This facility was set up to take care of lacerations, simple bone fractures, and injuries of that nature. He persisted to try to tell us what to do until I told a police officer to get him away from the ambulance and clear a path so the ambulance could get going to the hospital. We transported the young boy to the hospital, yet he never recovered from that injury.

*****

Since I worked the night shift, my shift was to end at 7:00 AM. One of the day-shift paramedics asked me to stay on because he was going to be late. Both paramedic units were at the hospital when we got dispatched. We used a ten-code system where information would be dispatched using this system. Examples were a 10-88, which means cardiac arrest; 10-29 means possible death, and so on. When we got this particular ten-code dispatch, we all looked at each other and said, "What is that?" We quickly looked it up and realized it was an aircraft down. We were responding to an area where the first aid squad would typically cancel paramedics en route to any call. We took a strategic move to get to this call. One paramedic unit took one route, and the other unit took another route. As we came up to the area, there was a man sitting on the side of the road who had blood on his shirt. We asked him what had happened, and he stated that he was the pilot of a single-engine plane, and they had crashed into the forest last night. He stated that the passenger was still at the crash scene and was hurt badly. One paramedic unit took care of the pilot, and the other unit went back into the forest with the police and firemen to find the passenger. Both men were brought to the hospital and survived their injuries. During this call, the first aid squad worked well with the paramedics, and it may have been a turning point to them accepting the fact that paramedics were there to help their patients, not take their patients away from them.

*****

When I was a paramedic student, I had a preceptor who instructed me to learn where everything in the medication box was located. I took the box, sat on a stretcher in the ER, and went through it over and over. Later that day, we had a cardiac arrest call, and the preceptor paramedics were asking me to hand them drugs from the medication box as they administered them. After the call, one paramedic said to me, "You did good."

*****

Most students that rotated on our shift were ready and eager to learn, yet one student, and I cannot remember his name for the life of me, was not that kind of student. As he was training with other paramedics, he got the reputation of being a know-it-all. When he arrived for our shift, I wanted him to understand that I would let him perform tasks as long as I felt he was capable of doing them. He entered our building, and I introduced myself, my partner, and the day-shift paramedics. He did not seem as enthusiastic as others, but everyone was different. I knew that he had been with other paramedics and should know the basics. I told him that we were going to check the equipment. We went out to the truck and got the two medication boxes, and I gave him one of the checklists we used. Keep in mind that I checked these boxes every shift I work, and I knew where the medication was located and when the expiration dates of each medication were. I gave him the box that was to be used first this shift, and I took the backup box. We brought them inside and began going through them. While I was halfway through checking my box, he closed the box he was checking. I asked him if he had checked for all the medication. He said that he had. I told him to return it to the truck and bring in the airway box so he could check that. When he returned, I again asked him if all the medication was in the box he checked.

He said, "I said I checked it. How many times are you going to ask me that?"

So I reached onto my pocket and pulled out a vial of morphine from the box he had checked and said to him, "If you checked the box, then why do I have a vial of morphine from your box?" He realized then that I was not going to accept his word or attitude. I told him to go get the medication box, handed him the "missing" morphine vial, and told him to check the box again.

The paramedic who worked the shift before us, who had also trained with us came up to me and said, "I am glad you never did that to me!"

I responded, "I never had the need to."

*****

Back in the day, we did not have GPS. We had paper maps, and with all the retirement villages that have so many small streets in them, responding out of our normal area driving could be a challenge. We also had a deer population issue, and at dusk and dawn, I cannot tell you how many units were involved with deer hits, yet I was never involved in any of them. We were getting a bite to eat, and we got a call in a neighboring town. We were moving along and went through this congested intersection during rush hour, and there was an S curve. The only thing that worried me about that curve, when navigating through it, was that there was a lake on one side of it right next to the road. We got close to the edge yet did not end up in the lake, but my partner thought we were going into the lake.

*****

When the hospital moved us from the first aid squad building to a modular building next door, it was great because we had space to keep our things, bunk beds, and closets to keep all our medical supplies. One day, a stray dog came around, and we started giving it water and food. We then took him in and named him Nitro. He stayed with us for a while until the director found out about it, and they moved him to a shelter. He was a glimmer of hope on those tough shifts when he would just snuggle up to you as if he knew you had a bad call.

Volunteer Ambulance (After Becoming a Nurse and Paramedic)

So my friend Debbie once again recruited me to join the volunteer first aid squad, and I volunteered close to twenty years to this first aid squad. Most times, we would be on the crew together unless one of us was working or had something else planned. There was a call of a car into a tree not far from the first aid building, so Debbie and I headed to the scene. When we got there, the car was literally torn in half, each side of it on the side of a tree. The young male had numerous life-threatening injuries. We got him on the stretcher with the help of the fire department and loaded him into the ambulance. He went into cardiac arrest, and we started chest compressions. We asked how far away the paramedics were and were told they would arrive in less than thirty seconds. Both the back door and the side door to the ambulance were open so they could get in the ambulance quickly, and one of the firemen would drive their truck to the hospital. The paramedic crew that responded was my husband and Debbie's mother. We continued CPR all the way to the hospital, yet he would be another young man who would not survive his injuries.

*****

We got dispatched to a car into a pole on one of the fairly busy streets in town. When we arrived, the woman was unresponsive, and both her legs were trapped underneath the dashboard. Since I am only five feet two inches tall, it was easiest for me to get in the back seat to hold her neck for stabilization while the firemen tried to cut the car apart to free the woman. Debbie placed a helmet on my head and covered us both with a blanket as the fire department went to work using the Jaws of Life and other tools. The paramedics arrived, and I gave them the information I knew up to that point, and they tried to treat the woman from the passenger side of the car. The fire department had removed the roof, the driver door, and pulled up the steering column away from her so we could try and get the woman, who weighed approximately three hundred pounds, out of the small car. She had broken both her femurs and was going into shock. There were trauma centers at this time, so they had requested a helicopter, and it was landing in the park nearby. The woman did recover, yet she had to live in a nursing home after.

*****

Debbie and I had a small consulting business and had an office in the downtown area. We had our first aid pagers on while we were at the office one day, and the tones for all five first aid squads in our town went off. The call was for a bus accident in the median of the Garden State Parkway, and our office was less than two minutes to the parkway, so off we headed up the parkway for about four miles. The bus was actually in the median embankment next to the parkway and stopped just shy of the guardrail and road beneath. There were ten people taken to nearby hospitals, yet no injuries were life-threatening. The other people who were not injured just wanted to know how they were going to get to Atlantic City to finish their day trip.

*****

It was a morning just before Christmas when I was out doing errands. It had snowed the night before, and the roads had snow on them, yet I was driving a Mustang, and those cars do not handle well in snow. The call came out for an infant not breathing. I headed toward the house since I knew that the ambulance crew would already be on their way to the call. As I slid through intersections, weaving my way to the small street, I saw the ambulance, which only had Debbie and a new EMT on it, heading toward the street where the call was. We ran into the house, loaded the baby into the back of the ambulance, and headed to the hospital because paramedics were not available at the time of the call. The child did not survive, yet Debbie said to me after the call, "I was never so glad to see your car turn the corner. I knew it was you because of the wreath on the car."

*****

So in early January 1996, New Jersey got a blizzard with tremendous winds. The plan was to bring our children to the first aid squad building since we were on duty, and most of our family members were *essential personnel* who also had to go to work. Some other first aid members did the same. Well, that plan ended up lasting a few days since the snow was intense. Debbie and I were going to go to the grocery store before it got too bad to get food and supplies for all those staying at the building. We got our supplies and, of course, got stuck in the snow outside of the grocery store. The fire department had to come and help get us out. The children loved the idea of sleeping over at the first aid building and actually kept themselves entertained by watching movies and building tents out of sheets and blankets. During that time, we did get a call for an elderly male who was not feeling well. Since the snow was coming down so fast, the fire department sent a fire truck ahead of us to plow the road so we could get to any calls. There was no way we could get a stretcher to the house from the street, so we had to place the elderly male on some blankets, place him on a Reeves stretcher, and actually slid him across the snow to the ambulance. It seemed like it took hours to get to the hospital because the roads were snow-covered, and the blizzard winds were blowing snow in every direction.

*****

At one point, I was the second lieutenant on the first aid squad, so I had a radio that I could take home. I was home cleaning the house one afternoon, and I was in the middle of vacuuming. When I turned the vacuum off, my radio and pager were going crazy with dispatches. I heard there had been a shooting in town, and they were dispatching all ambulance squads (we had five different squads in our town), along with the paramedics, the police, the police SWAT team, and police K-9 units. Both the police SWAT team and the K-9 units were in training that day and ready to respond instantly. This happened in the middle of the afternoon and schools were in the process of busing students to their homes from numerous schools. The school buses were all held at the schools, and those that had already left the schools were rerouted away from the neighborhood involved. I was on the opposite side of town, but I got in my car and headed to the first aid squad. We had three ambulances at the time, and as I turned onto the street where the first aid squad building was located, the second ambulance passed me heading to the scene. I got to the building and got on the third ambulance responding to the scene. They were staging emergency vehicles down the block from the incident. As we were responding, this was still an active shooter incident, so there were a lot of unknowns. When we came up to the scene, Debbie was on the first ambulance in, and they already had a patient in the back of the ambulance with gunshot wounds and the paramedics present. His condition was critical at that time, and they were preparing him for a helicopter ride to the trauma center. I could see there was a person on a front lawn already covered with a sheet. The police officers, SWAT team members, and the K-9 units were trying to find the shooter and piece together the events that had taken place just moments before. The paramedics wanted me to drive their vehicle to the helicopter landing zone because they were both going in the ambulance with the patient. The only problem was that the paramedic's vehicle was parked a block away opposite where the ambulances were. A police officer had to escort me down the street toward the paramedic vehicle while passing gun shell casings all over the road. At this time, my husband, who was the SWAT team commander saw me and was upset that I was there. The patient was transported to the landing zone and placed in the helicopter to go to the trauma center. He succumbed to his injuries and was the fourth victim to die in this shooting spree. Less than two months later, the town had another shooting spree where the shooter killed five people and injured two others before taking his own life.

*****

Our first aid squad and the paramedics got dispatched to a house for an unresponsive patient. When we arrived, there was only one small narrow path from the front door to the back bedroom of the house where the patient was. The house was so hot, with a nasty smell throughout. The debris in this house was over five feet tall, and it was everywhere. We could not bring a stretcher in, nor could we carry a person through this narrow path. We called for the fire department, and they had to cut out the window because they were all nailed shut, and we had to put the patient on a long backboard and slide her out the window to the stretcher we had set up outside. I do not know the status of that woman, yet years later, the house was knocked down.

*****

Another call we went on was for an unresponsive male in his house. When we arrived, we found the male in the back bedroom, and the house had been closed up for days. The smell coming from the front door was so rancid, yet we had to get in there and get this man out of the house for the paramedics who had set up in our ambulance. We transported him to the hospital, where he later died, and it took hours to clean and air out the ambulance from that smell that just would not go away.

*****

I was off from work one day, heading out to do some errands, and one of the other first aid squads in town got a call for a possible death. Since the crews of the day shift are usually staffed with only two EMTs, I headed toward the scene. When I got there, the police were outside an apartment complex with a set of stairs heading to the second floor. I went into the landing at the bottom of the stairs and noted the smell of a decomposing body. There was no need for a first aid squad at this time. The police had received a call of concern from someone since they had not heard from the woman in days. The middle-aged woman was found hanging in her apartment.

*****

When Superstorm Sandy hit the Jersey Shore on October 29, 2012, it hit parts of our town extremely hard. Although the iconic picture of the roller coaster in the ocean after the storm was not part of our town, we did have property on that barrier reef as well as many houses that are located directly on the shores of the bay. The water surge that occurred with this storm did an immense amount of damage that would take years to rebuild.

The National Guard was called in, and we offered our first aid squad building as a housing area for the approximately fifty individuals who were deployed to help our town. We had a big meeting room upstairs and a large basement, so there was plenty of room to set up cots. There were all kind of vehicles, and radio equipment were brought in, and they set up camp so to say. Local restaurants delivered food three times a day to both our building as well as our firehouse a few blocks away. The firehouse served as a transfer station for those who had to leave their homes and be placed in shelters. As the weeks after the storm went on, it was getting closer to the holidays of Thanksgiving, Christmas, and the New Year. The local fire department sold Christmas trees each year, and this year was no different as people tried to get back to some kind of normalcy. We asked them if they could deliver a Christmas tree to the first aid building so we could decorate it for the National Guard personnel. They were very gracious and brought us a beautiful tree that we put in the ambulance bay, and Debbie and I proceeded to decorate it. We felt that just did not seem like enough to thank them for all that they had done for our community, so we made gift bags for each of them and put them under the Christmas tree. The commander of the unit received orders that their assignment was to end a few days before Christmas, so each of them got their Christmas gift bags, which they were very appreciative of, and more importantly, they all got to spend time with their families during the holiday season.

Correctional Facility Audits and Technical Assist Visits

I was on various audit teams that went into jails and prisons nationwide to verify that the facility was compliant with specific standards regarding the function, care, and safety issues as they related to staff and detainees. Since I am a nurse, I concentrated on the standards that pertained to the medical, dental, and psychological needs and services for the detainees. Audits would have mandatory standards that must have 100 percent compliance and essential standards that had a 90 percent compliance to pass the inspection. For all the audits I went on, we were there to gather information, review, and witness policies and procedures in place and would report back to the governing agency where a decision to pass the facility was determined. To anyone who has worked in a hospital, it is equivalent to a visit from the Joint Commission and can be nerve-wracking for some. We knew that the facility may have tried to find out any information on each of the auditors before we arrived. One warden commented to me that he saw that I had published articles in a jail magazine, and I told him that I had and that one of the issues I had been published in was on his magazine rack in his office. I found that each auditor has one issue that is of utmost concern for them no matter what standard they are reviewing, such as chemical control, cleanliness, recordkeeping, and provision of services to name a few.

In a jail in New Mexico, the facility had approximately three times the number of people the facility was designed for. Surprisingly, it was very clean, and the detainees we spoke to did not have any complaints of not having enough space, and there were few fights reported. The audit team consisted of two male auditors and me. We went into the super max dorm where the detainees were charged with the most serious crimes, such as murder, rape, and aggravated assault. We each spoke to a group of detainees within the housing unit, and when we came back out into the hallway, one of the other auditors said that a detainee asked him if the detainee could come into my group because I was better-looking than the male auditor.

At another audit, I was taking a break outside the main front door to the administrative area of the facility when all of a sudden, staff members came running past me stating, "There is someone on the roof." The reason they were running to check the outside is because only about two hundred feet from the facility was an interstate highway where someone could have been there waiting for a detainee who may have escaped. After a few tense moments, it was determined that it was a contractor on the roof who had not checked in with the security staff, so when the securing staff saw someone on the roof in the camera, they were not aware that he was up there working. The next day, while at the same facility, I was accompanying the nurse doing a medication pass in one of the dorms. All of a sudden, I heard the sound of boots running and saw the numerous officers running toward our direction, so I just moved against the wall so they could rush by us. They were heading to another dorm of a fight in progress, and after it was taken care of, one of the officers stopped and said to me, "You are some auditor…you are always where there is something going on."

*****

I was asked to go to a facility in Colorado to do a pre-audit visit on the medical department where I was there to identify any issues, offer suggestions to fix any issues, and prepare the medical unit staff for their upcoming audit. The security staff administration and compliance officer thought that there may be some issues that needed to be addressed and wanted those issues corrected prior to the actual audit visit. For the most part, policies and procedures were appropriate to the standards and were being followed by the staff. The correctional facility environment was extremely focused on safety and the well-being of both detainees and staff. Contraband was an ongoing issue in all facilities, and some contraband could be used to cause harm to someone—such as, medications, sharp objects, and chemicals within the facility. At this facility, I had an issue with the storage and tracking stocks of narcotic medication. The issue was not within each of the medication carts that were taken to each dorm to administer medication to detainees since the narcotics in the medication carts had tracking sheets for each narcotic and had a double locking system. The issue was with the replacement of stock narcotics that were kept in a cabinet in the room where the medication carts were locked when not in use. They were double locked, as required, yet there was no accountability as to the number of narcotics in this cabinet. I explained my concern to the warden in a meeting and told him that since these narcotics were not being counted every shift, then someone could take some of these narcotics, and it may go unnoticed and be almost impossible to track back to when they may have been taken. The warden and the compliance officer understood my issue and were not happy when I explained that I felt that I could get some of these narcotics out of that unit without the staff being aware. The warden advised me to go back to the medical unit, advised them of my concerns, and explained how to correct this issue immediately. The reason I understood that this warden was serious about this issue was because he told me that if this issue was not corrected by morning, that I had permission from him to take some of those narcotics with the compliance officer present and remove them from the medical unit to prove my point. Luckily, the staff corrected the issue, so I did not have to prove that someone could steal narcotics from their unit.

*****

At a facility in Virginia, Debbie and I were asked to visit the medical department for an evaluation of their medical unit, policies, and procedures, and to prepare the staff for an upcoming accreditation audit. The facility was only one year old and built with the medical unit being very spacious and had a full medical, dental, and mental health staff. We found that there were many sick call slips that had not been evaluated. There was a whiteboard with detainee names and diagnoses on it in the main area of the medical department, and then there was the issue of the physician's examination room. I walked into the physician's examination room and almost fell over because there were needles, syringes, and implements such as scissors, tweezers, and scalpel handles all over the counter. Keep in mind that this is a jail and all these items can become potential weapons if someone wanted to take them. We brought this to the attention of the health service administrator and the facility captain, who was our contact person, and the room was immediately cleaned, and all those items were locked in cabinets. The next day, the facility was supplying lunch for the nurses for nurses' week, and the number of correctional officers that told us that they heard that the physician's examination room was clean was staggering since my thought was that the officers are there to protect all people within the facility, and if they knew this room was in that condition, why didn't they bring it to someone's attention prior to us arriving?

*****

In a facility in Florida, the audit team was comprised of three women—one from Colorado, one from Virginia, and I was from New Jersey—and the facility compliance officer was also a woman. The warden was a quiet young man, yet the rest of his administrative staff was so funny. They kept telling me that I reminded them of Ms. Veto from the movie *My Cousin Vinnie* since I had the Jersey accent, big hair, and talked fast. We asked the warden at the end of the audit if he had been worried about having an all-women audit team, and he told us that he had no worries about it. That is, when all three of us said, almost in unison, "We were." The administrative staff told me I could not drive the rental car since I was from New Jersey, and they said we drive crazy. We were going to pull a joke on them on the last day when we drove in by placing a palm tree branch in the grill of the car, but of course, we did not pass one palm leaf along the way to the facility that morning.

*****

Every auditor has that one issue that they will always focus in on no matter what facility they are in. I worked with one auditor many times throughout the years, and his main issue was chemicals and caustics. If there was any type of spray bottle anywhere in the facility and he sees it, he would ask the officer to track the bottle back to the location where it was distributed from since cleaning fluids are not kept within housing units so they cannot be used to harm anyone. On the first day of the audit visit, the facility administrative staff took the audit team on a tour of the entire facility. We were near the kitchen area and the delivery loading dock when there was another door to another room. The facility administrative staff representative said the room was used by the county employees for storage, which was the size of about a four-car garage. This auditor wanted to see this room since the room was part of the building structure. When they opened the door, I thought this auditor would have a heart attack because there were paint cans, gas cans, landscaping equipment, tools, and other chemicals all over this room. The facility did not believe that it was their responsibility since it was maintained and used by county workers, yet the auditor explained that because this room is within the walls of the facility, the standards on chemical and caustics did pertain, and of course, chemical and caustics is a mandatory standard. He agreed to give them until the next day to correct the issue. All I know is that some of the staff looked very tired the next day, and when we went back to that room the next day, there was literally nothing in that room except empty shelves, so they did not fail that standard.

Some of the standards are broad in scope, and that standard may pertain to more than one auditor based on the areas we would focus on. For instance, since I focused on the medical department, I would check anything that dealt with the sharps and key control standard that is actually another standard. At one facility, I went to the medical department and asked the health service administrator to count the sharps, including any needles, syringes, scalpels, ring cutter to mention a few. We were going through the count, and there was one scalpel not accounted for. This was also a mandatory standard, and the audit could come to a halt if this issue was not rectified immediately. After about twenty minutes, it was determined that a nurse practitioner had used a scalpel for a procedure earlier that day, yet no one had signed the sharp count, so it was corrected. I went back to the medical unit the next day and did a sharp count with a day-shift nurse, and the insulin syringe count was off. I contacted the health service administrator and voiced my concern, then the search was on for the missing syringe. They finally tracked it back to the night-shift nurse who had to give an insulin injection on someone new to the facility because their blood sugar was elevated when they arrived, yet that nurse did not sign that needle out on the sharp count. The day-shift nurse was counseled because she should have caught the missing syringe during the morning change-of-shift count.

In the jail where I was the health service administrator, the warden felt so strong about the safety of sharps in his facility that our policy and procedure was to have a nurse and an officer do the sharps count every shift.

*****

In one facility, the warden had staff members cook a big lunch for us and all the staff one day. This was a smaller facility, and they were very close-knit. People brought in so much food I could not believe it, yet it was a very nice gesture and saved time for us because the only place we could go to have lunch was about forty-five minutes away from the facility. I remember one staff member told us that a dish she made was *really hot* and to avoid it if we did not like spicy food. We had everything from salads to fried chicken to gumbo to desserts.

In Louisiana, the warden was going to have lunch—which consisted of corn bread, coleslaw, fried alligator, and alligator gumbo—brought in to the facility for the audit team. I asked for a lot of ketchup and a diet Pepsi since I was not sure if I would like it. I told them it tasted like chicken from a lake, and the next day when we were driving to go out to lunch, the warden said, "Roadkill," and I responded, "I do not want it for lunch."

In Colorado, a mandatory standard that dealt with every detainee receiving a physical assessment within fourteen days of arrival was in jeopardy. When I reviewed the audit file the medical staff presented for the audit, there were a number of charts where this standard was not met, which gave me much concern. So I had the correctional staff run off a list of those detainees who had arrived over the last two months, and I highlighted twenty names for the medical unit to pull for my review. They were able to provide me with ten charts since the other names had either been released or their charts were not in the file cabinet indicating that the chart was with a provider. I told the medical unit to pick out five more charts for me to review. Out of the fifteen charts I reviewed, only eight charts were compliant with the standard. I discussed my findings with the other auditors, and a call had to be made to the governing body to advise the fact that this facility was not meeting this mandatory standard. The lead auditor advised the facility that the audit would end and that this visit would become a technical assist visit and that the facility would have to reapply for a new audit to maintain their accreditation.

During another audit, when I was interviewing detainees in different dorms, I got many complaints that they were putting in sick call slips for medical, dental, or mental health services, and they were not hearing back from the medical department. This troubled me because this was the primary way that detainees request nonemergency medical services and requests. I decided to try a bit of a test to see how the sick call slips are handled from the detainee dorms to the medical department. I wrote out a sick call slip that said, "I have chest pain...contact Susan, the auditor," and went to the female dorm and asked one of the detainees to place this sick call request in the box later in the evening. I could not put the medical request slip in the box myself because the officer would have observed this and contacted the medical department. The next day, I was out in the facility going to different areas since I was talking to staff members from the social service department, the religious program, the education department, and the recreation officer when I heard over the radio that a member of the medical staff was looking for "Susan, the auditor." I knew then that they had received the sick call slip and was following the instructions to contact me. The facility staff nurses finally caught up with me in their medical unit, and I asked them what evaluation they would do with a patient with chest pain, and they described everything they would do correctly.

Correctional Health Care and Nursing Conference Presentations

I have presented sessions for over twenty years at state and national conferences on various nursing-related topics. I began wearing pink slippers during some of these conferences since I was not used to wearing high heels, and at times, I had to dash from one session to another.

People associate me with my pink slippers. So one year, a few of my close correctional nursing friends and I did a session celebrating nurses, and it had the title "My Pink Slippers." We all wore our pink slippers and crowns and provided all participants small candles to hold up as we all sang the song "You Raise Me Up."

I have met some incredible people over the years and have made lifelong friends with a few. We would teach sessions together, be on committees together, be board members, and work on tasks forces for special projects related to nursing care. We loved to do sessions that were engaging and thought-provoking for our audiences. We would design scenarios to demonstrate the topic that we were discussing. One session even had participants moving around the room in a conga line. A dear friend Margaret, who is looking down from heaven on us now, was the "queen" of nursing education and always had a smile that just kept on going. During one session, she wore a large biohazard bag over her clothing and said to me, "I have been waiting years to do this."

*****

One year, we were going to do a hands-on session regarding medical emergencies. I recruited many friends—some who moderated the scenarios, some who dressed in orange T-shirts and were made up to have injuries so participants would rotate through as a group through different stations. Margaret had always wanted to do this session with me, yet when I got approved, she had already gone to heaven, so we dedicated the session to her.

*****

I have done sessions with some incredible physicians who are not only extremely knowledgeable and have résumés that read like novels but remain down to earth. I presented a few sessions with one physician who had worked in both ED and correctional settings like me. After one such session, another physician who had attended the class came up to us and asked me how long we had been working together. We both laughed and told him we have never worked together in either setting. During another session with this physician, he wanted me to play act the part of an inmate. So during lunch, I changed into a white T-shirt and jeans. People usually wear casual business attire during the conferences, so I got some strange looks as I was going through the hallways toward the class, and a few people who knew me did not even recognize me. The physician was doing a session on back pain and was describing how to determine if a patient had legitimate back pain issues. He stated his session, and I was in the audience when he wanted his "patient" to come to the front of the room.

I stood up and said, "Doc, I hope you can give me some of that cotton medicine," and the audience laughed. He then wanted me to lie down on one of the tables in front of the room. I was just praying the table would not fall down as he described techniques to determine back pain issues. We did another presentation entitled "The 3:00 AM Wake-Up Call" that focused on the communication skills needed between nurses and physicians.

*****

We invited Mother Antonia, to speak at an early breakfast session during one of our conferences and had the pleasure to meet her in person and throw a small reception for her in a condo we had rented in Las Vegas. She was a woman who grew up in Beverly Hills, and after her children were grown, she became a nun and moved to Tijuana, Mexico, and actually lived in a prison while providing spiritual guidance to those imprisoned there. Her words were truly inspirational, and she was kind enough to autograph each copy of the book written about her for each of my friends during the reception.

*****

When I am traveling to these conferences, my suitcase and carry-on always has little gifts for participants in my sessions. I usually have a handout for the session, and I would put a sticker on the back of it to designate who had won a prize. The prizes were always given out at the end of the session. I have been doing this for so many years that I have seen people come into the session, be given the handout, and flip it over to see if they may have one before ever sitting down.

We have attended and arranged some fun gatherings over the years and always enjoyed the chance to spend time with friends who we would see only once or twice a year.

*****

Early in my correctional health-care career as a nurse, I obtained the certified correctional health-care professional (CCHP) certification. That led me to also obtain the advanced certification (CCHP-A), and at one time, there were approximately twenty-five people in the United States who had obtained this certification. I was asked to be on the task force to develop the specialty certification for registered nurses (CCHP-RN) to include identifying tasks specific to correctional health-care nurses, writing examination questions, and developing and providing review courses for this certification. I am very proud of obtaining these certifications, and all of them remain current.

Nursing All the Time

Debbie and I have traveled many times on airline flights, but two in particular were a bit more eventful than we wanted. On one occasion, we were flying to a conference for correctional health-care workers. I had worked a twelve-hour shift before boarding the plane and was tired. I usually do not wear a coat, yet I had one on since it was frigid outside, and the only time I am cold is when I am tired. I quickly started my nap as the plane took off, and sometime later, I remember hearing this scream, and in that instant, I thought, *I don't remember seeing any young children boarding the plane.* In the next second, Debbie hit me on the arm and said, "Come on." We both went toward the back of the plane where a man was unconscious in his seat. Of course, he had on layers of clothing under his jacket. I felt a pulse, yet it was very slow. As I tried to get the layers of clothing off the man, Debbie asked the flight attendant if they had any medical equipment on board, including an automated external defibrillator (AED).

The flight attendant looked like she was going to faint and said, "Yes, we have one, but I have never used it."

Debbie told her to get any equipment they had including the AED and oxygen. The man began to be more alert, yet he looked like he was going to vomit. Keep in mind that we are in the back of the plane, in the window seat, and the man weighed about 250 pounds and was elderly. Debbie asked the man's wife if he had any medical conditions, any allergies, or was on any medication, yet did not get much information since we later found out she had Alzheimer's and had a bad memory. Other passengers kept an eye on her and offered to help us if we needed anything. The only thought going through both of our minds was if this man went into cardiac arrest, we would have to get him to the front of the plane where there would be room to do CPR. The man gradually awoke and realized something had happened yet was concerned for his wife. The flight attendant while all this was going on told the pilot about the situation. They decided to make an emergency landing so the man could be brought to a local hospital for evaluation since we still had over two hours to our destination. The man looked down and saw that his coat and sweater had been removed and looked at me. I told him that even though I had just met him, I was the one who undressed him. The other passengers chuckled and realized that he was awake and talking. The man was concerned that his son was going to pick him and his wife up at the airport and might be worried if he and his wife did get off the plane anywhere other than their original destination. I told him that the hospital staff would get in contact with his son, and arrangements could be made once the man was evaluated. We made an unscheduled landing, and the ambulance was already there waiting for us to arrive. We helped the man down the aisle since there were no way we, even with the ambulance crew, would be able to carry him to the front of the plane. As we got to the steps of the plane, Debbie was in front of the man going down the steps backward, and I was behind him.

Debbie said to me, "Hold on to him."

I knew she was telling me that he was getting pale again and might pass out. We got him safely down the steps, put him on the ambulance stretcher as the ambulance crew asked us if we were going to the hospital with him. After we told them "No, we are not going with the man to the hospital," we gave them a quick report, placed his wife in the front of the ambulance, and off they went. We got back into our seats and started what I call the "Susan and Debbie Show," where we go back and forth to decide who brought on this medical emergency. I told Debbie that this happens when we fly together since I have flown many other times and never had any medical emergencies happen during my flights. There was a man in the seat in front of us who looked back at us between the seats. He was wearing airline apparel, and I asked him if he was a pilot. He told us that yes, he was a pilot, so I asked him if he wanted us on his plane, and he responded, "I don't think so."

Then I said to him, "If you got sick on your plane, would you want us there?" and he said, "Yes." This unscheduled landing made us late to the connecting airport, and a few other people had also

SUSAN LAFFAN

missed their connecting flights. While we stood in line to get to the ticket counter, many of the people who were on that plane thanked us for helping the man. When we got up to the counter, one of the other passengers, who was still in line, yelled, "You should upgrade them to first class since they just saved that man's life," and the girl at the counter simply said, "Their tickets are not for first class."

*****

On another flight returning home from a conference in Las Vegas, the flight was already delayed taking off due to mechanical problems, and people were getting tired of waiting. We saw an older lady in a wheelchair among others in the line to preboard. Once in the air, we heard the announcement we dread.

"If there is any medical professional on board, please make yourself known to a flight attendant."

Debbie and I did a quick scan of the plane, and no one was putting on their light, so we let them know we were both emergency department nurses. They escorted us toward the back of the plane, and there was the same lady we saw earlier in the wheelchair having trouble breathing. We asked the crew for oxygen, blood pressure cuff, and a stethoscope. As I took the woman's vitals and listened to her lungs, there was very little air movement. I looked up and wondered where Debbie went. Just as she came back, she told me that we could make an unscheduled landing, or we could be a priority landing to our original destination, yet that option was over one hour away. Debbie saw the look on my face and said, "Okay, I guess we are going down." The pilot made an announcement regarding the unscheduled landing, and one of the passengers started to complain to the flight attendant. So we told him to ask that passenger if it were their mother who was sick, wouldn't they want us to make the stop for the sick passenger? Debbie went back up the aisle, and when she returned, she told me that the flight crew had moved some passengers around so we could move the woman closer to the front of the plane. Unlike the other man we helped in the plane, this woman was only about one hundred pounds, so we began to move her down the aisle as the plane was leaning downward, and her legs buckled under her, so Debbie and I lifted her and carried her the rest of the way down the aisle. As we got to the row of seats, I looked up, and all the flight attendants were already wearing their seat belts with a scared look on their faces since we were about to land. We barely got the woman into the seat and put on her seat belt, and we landed. The ambulance crew came on board and took the woman to the hospital. We were standing in the front area by the door with the flight attendants, and they said, "Now we have another issue." I asked them if someone else was sick, and they told us that no one else was sick, yet this flight crew was now going to be over the flying time allowed. They said it would take hours to get another flight crew, and the pilot decided to just continue the flight as planned. As you can imagine, some of the passengers were not happy with all the delays, but in the end, no one died on the plane. Later, I asked Debbie where she went, and she said she was talking to the doctor over the radio in the cockpit. This event happened before they locked all cockpits on flights. Debbie also told me that when she went to talk to the doctor on the radio, she told him we were emergency department nurses, and the doctor's response was "Well, I wish there was a doctor on board." Debbie then said to the doctor, "Well, there isn't," and the pilot gave Debbie the thumbs-up sign. Debbie and I had no other experiences on any planes together, yet just last year, Debbie was flying home, and a young lady passed out. Of course, I had to remind Debbie that it had to be her that brought on sick people in planes since I was not there for that event, and we had a good laugh.

*****

One of my dear friends was a correctional physician and had also worked in an emergency room, so we always talked about stories we had at the conventions we both presented at. I told him about my airplane stories, and while we were returning from another conference, a group of us traveling, who were all nurses, figured we would joke with our physician friend. We knew that we would be landing at our destination before he was boarding his plane, so we called him and told him that we were in an airplane with a woman who was in labor and about to deliver. He was ready to talk us through it when we all started laughing and told him it was a joke.

*****

While I was working outside in the Florida heat, I heard someone say, "Are you okay?" so I looked around the corner and saw a middle-aged woman on the verge of passing out. Not only is it hot in Florida, yet the sun adds an extreme heat that people who visit do not always take in to account as they are walking around. I told her to sit down on the ground and lean against a support wall while her family watched. I only brought lunch to work about five times in the year I worked there, and I had brought a cooler with ice water and ice packs that day. I went and got the ice packs and had the woman hold one on her forehead, and I placed others on her neck. I had her sit there for about fifteen minutes when she told me she felt much better. She was no longer sweaty, and the pink color had returned to her face. I had the family go get their car and turn on the air-conditioning while I assisted the woman to get up slowly and lean on the supporting wall. After she got in to the air-conditioned care, she asked if she could keep the ice packs since they made her feel so much better, and of course, I told her she could keep them. Her sister gave me a big hug and thanked me for helping her sister when "she did not look good," as she described the event.

*****

We would have daily briefings at one job I was working at that provided tourist attractions. I asked one of the managers if I could speak to the group for about fifteen minutes regarding the topic of heat exhaustion since we were at the beginning of the summer. Some of the managers would simply say to us every day, "Drink a lot of water." I wanted to explain the signs and symptoms of heat exhaustion not only to the people I worked with, but also to those customers who were in one of our attractions. He allowed me to talk to the group on a Saturday morning before we all went to our respected posts. I had many people come up to me after that talk and compliment me on giving them valuable information.

One coworker said to me, "I used to run a Fortune 500 company, and that was one of the best presentations I have ever heard. And certainly the best one I have heard at this company."

Another employee came up to me and said, "I have felt some of those things you described, and now I know to watch out for them, thanks."

Other employees would joke and say, "It is more than just drinking water."

It felt good to provide those I was working with some valuable information that may keep them from getting ill.

*****

When my son was coming to visit Key West one summer, I booked a trip for all of us, my husband and my neighbor to go on a day trip to the Dry Tortugas National Park, which is seventy miles west of Key West in the Gulf of Mexico. I thought that would be a great birthday gift for him since his birthday is in August. We headed to the ferry pier early in the day to check in and board the boat for the two-and-half-hour trip to the Dry Tortugas and had breakfast on board. We chatted the entire way with stories of me as a nurse, my son the fireman, my husband the police officer, and our neighbor the nurse, who also came on this trip. My husband and I had been on this trip before, yet for the others, it was their first time. When we docked at the island, we decided to walk through the fort first before having lunch or going swimming and snorkeling. About five minutes into our walk around the fort, I noticed the AED hanging on the wall near the entrance on the first floor. We took pictures of the fort and headed to the beach to find a place to put our stuff down and get some lunch. After lunch, my husband and son were going to go snorkeling. I was standing at the water edge taking pictures of them, and as I was returning to the area we had put all our things, I heard a man in the water yell, "This guy is unconscious, and I don't think he is breathing." People went running into the water to help get the person out of the water. I yelled to my family and pointed in the direction of where the people were, and I ran up the beach and down the wall that surrounded the fort since the people had lifted this man onto the moat wall. When they laid him down on his back, I could tell that he was not breathing as his skin tone had turned a deep blue. My husband and son quickly joined me, and we began CPR as I told the people around us to notify the park rangers. When a park ranger arrived, I told him to bring any medical equipment such as oxygen and the AED. Shortly after starting CPR, I told my son to turn the man to his side, and he gave him a modified Heimlich maneuver, and the man expelled a lot of water and undigested food. The family and friends were still on the other side of the fort at this time, unaware of the events. The man's family and friends told the park rangers that he did not feel good when they were snorkeling, and he was going to return to the beach after they arrived where we were located. I overheard the wife tell the park ranger that the man had high blood pressure yet did not take any medication and had no allergies. I asked the park rangers if a helicopter had been called, and they told me that yes, one had been called, yet there was no estimated time of arrival. We were able to move the man off the wall, all the time continuing CPR with my son, my husband, and two other men assisting us, rotating turns doing compressions since we were in the hot sun, in the middle of the day. This continued on for over one hour while we waited for the helicopter to arrive. I gave the flight team a report of the events that happened, the man's medical history, and that the AED only had one time when it delivered a defibrillator shock to the man. After the helicopter left, there was only about thirty minutes until the boat was to leave the island for the return trip back to Key West. To say that we were exhausted after this event would be an understatement. The man did pass away at the hospital, yet I knew we had all done everything we could to revive him. One of the boat crew members was also my neighbor and told me to let him know if I wanted to take another day trip, he would arrange it, in gratitude for all that we did for this man. I said thank you, yet I have not been back to the Dry Tortugas National Park since that day.

I continue to take these experiences and use them to educate others while using one of my most used statements: "If you are prepared for the worst that could happen to your patient, then you can handle anything else."

As this book comes to an end, I am grateful for all the wonderful people I have met and worked with through this journey of my nursing and paramedic career, and thank you for being part of these memories. Thank you for what you do or have done every day to help people. You may never truly know the number of lives you have touched.

ABOUT THE AUTHOR

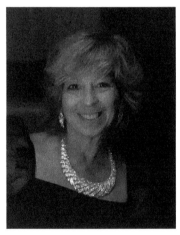 Susan Laffan—RN, CCHP-RN, CCHP-Advanced—has been a registered nurse for the last forty years working in emergency departments, critical care units, correctional facilities, and in the field as a paramedic. She is the wife of Tom and mother to Thomas and Katie, whom she is very proud of. Susan has had over forty nursing-related articles published, wrote a chapter in a correctional nursing textbook, and has provided educational sessions at conferences for twenty years at the state and national level

Susan has been an expert witness for lawyers nationwide regarding nursing care within correctional facilities and has been an accreditation auditor completing on-site surveys in jails and prisons nationwide.

Susan has also been a board member, task force member, or chairperson for correctional-related national organizations and was on the inception task force to develop and write questions for the Certified Correctional Health Professional RN certification examination.

CPSIA information can be obtained
at www.ICGtesting.com
Printed in the USA
BVHW091332030522
635995BV00049B/2401